Research Me

Research Me

GOD, BODY, ILLNESS

• • •

A book about taking accountability for and ownership of your health and wellness.

Sindy P. Heard

© 2017 Sindy P. Heard
All rights reserved.

ISBN: 1979990948
ISBN 13: 9781979990943
Library of Congress Control Number: 2017914668
CreateSpace Independent Publishing Platform
North Charleston, South Carolina

Preface

• • •

I WROTE THIS FROM THE perspective of my own personal journey in finding a fix for an illness. I wanted desperately to feel better so, I discovered that by identifying the root cause, I could find a solution. Quickly, I began investigating what my illness could be, thinking that a doctor could tell me what it was/is, only to be passed around from doctor to doctor. Frustrated, I did not get anywhere, only my condition got worse. In the end, I began to realized that health care is not care; it is just a wall that I encountered. Sadly, it did not get me closer to healing my illness. Looking at the bigger picture, I saw that I was not alone. I saw that others out there, were not being healed. Instead, they were being unnecessarily prescribed medications that covered them like a bandage, only masking the true issues of their illnesses. Their illnesses worsened, causing additional problems. Enough is enough, I thought! I did not want to go down the same path as everyone else, only to fill my body with medications that doctors were quick to prescribe, ultimately, I knew that was not the solution. I took my illness into my own hands accepting full accountability for myself, and wanting to feel better again. I knew that I could possibly find answers through the internet, knowing it is populated with tons of good and helpful information. I knew I had to weed through a lot of nonfactual information along the way. I also saw that other people would post things on the internet trying to find others with similar symptoms and illnesses.

As a spiritual individual, I didn't see a connection of why people gets sick in the first place. I then realized because of free will, we go through consequences we set for ourselves through many bad choices and decisions we make in our life, and by the environmental pollutants that we are all exposed to. I saw that everything was out there to be researched. So much information was at my fingertips. I was excited by the knowledge I was getting and becoming more positive about finding a solution.

Sadly, I see that our health-care system is not getting better and is not really affordable anymore. Currently, with all the government restraints put on health care, physicians of all types are being forced into certain guidelines and restrictions. The most knowledgeable doctors will eventually become obsolete, leaving the doctors who are corrupted by the system.

I hope this story I took to healing in Research Me; God, body, and illness, inspires people to research as well. We are our own teachers, and we can achieve anything we want to in life; we just have to start somewhere. As Simon Sinek, an author and motivational speaker, says, "There are only two ways to influence human behavior: you can manipulate it or you can inspire it." Sinek also says, "People don't buy what you do; they buy why you do it. And what you do simply proves what you believe."[1] I think this is an amazing principle to follow in any situation. Be a leader. Take a stand. Enjoy Research Me, a personal story to healing, pact with information that could be helpful in researching your own illnesses.

---

1 Simonsinek.com / startwithwhy.com/simon-sinek/© Simon Sinek INC. P.O. Box 230006, New York, NY, 10023, United States

Contents

Preface · v

Chapter 1   Discovering "it" · 1
Chapter 2   First-Aid Kit · 4
Chapter 3   Observations · 9
Chapter 4   My Backstory · 12
Chapter 5   Root Cause · 20
Chapter 6   Building an Action Plan · · · · · · · · · · · · · · · · · 23
Chapter 7   Questions Confirmed · · · · · · · · · · · · · · · · · · 25
Chapter 8   Healthy Heart · 28
Chapter 9   Bacteria and Virus · 37
Chapter 10 Look Up in the Air! It's Superbug! · · · · · · · · · · 41
Chapter 11 The Drug Effect · 44
Chapter 12 The Drug's Life · 46
Chapter 13 Cells · 48
Chapter 14 Deoxyribonucleic Acid (DNA) · · · · · · · · · · · · 53
Chapter 15 Immune System · 56
Chapter 16 Immune Response System · · · · · · · · · · · · · · 58
Chapter 17 Autoimmunity & Causes · · · · · · · · · · · · · · · 64
Chapter 18 Molecular-Level Autoimmunity · · · · · · · · · · · 67
Chapter 19 Causes of Autoimmune Disease · · · · · · · · · · · 69

Chapter 20	Micronutrients	71
Chapter 21	Journaling	73
Chapter 22	First Milk Benefits	75
Chapter 23	Health and Sleep	76
Chapter 24	Diacom	77
Chapter 25	Breath of Air	80
Chapter 26	Blood Work and Testing	82
	Final Thoughts	93
	Acknowledgments	97
	Author Biography	99
	Personal Journal	101

CHAPTER 1
Discovering "it"

• • •

AT SOME POINTS IN OUR lives, we all have imbalances inside our bodies that happen, things like exposer to viruses or harmful bacteria that take their toll on us. Around the globe, but especially in America, people want easy fixes for their illnesses. They want a magic pill that masks the pain, so they don't experience the discomforting feelings of any illness that takes away any quality of life.

We all should take a proactive approach to discovering the true causes of our illnesses, however. We must focus on finding the cause before treating any illness with any type of prescription drug. We must become more in tune with our own bodies, and know and understand what our bodies are trying to alert us to when we experience those pains. We have to ask ourselves whether it is a chronic, or an abnormal pain. Maybe it's an acute pain, or a dull pain or a localized pain. Pain is the body's way of saying, "Help me out. There is something going on that needs attention."

People are becoming too apathetic to research the problem themselves, and this is becoming a serious problem. When we just utilize doctors, we only get a magic pill that covers up the root problem like a bandage would a wound. It does not really solve the problem at all, it just masks it. In my experience, most of the doctors I saw would not take additional steps towards finding the root cause, "because they have too many patients", as one said to me. My belief is that the medical industry is focused on making money, not training doctors to solve health issues. This can't be the way it is supposed to be. Doctor's should be educated to find real solutions to treat the root causes of illnesses their patients get. The way it is now, only is getting the patient to return for more meds. I don't know about you, but I don't want to spend my life in doctors' offices, and all I end up getting is a prescription, that I may or may not need to take for the rest of my years.

Because of this, I feel that it is so important to take accountability and responsibility for our own health, and get to know how our body reacts to certain things, and know what our bodies' signals are when it comes to illnesses, or disease. Research is the starting point to most things; why not to our health?

Chronic pain is pain that lasts for a long time.

Acute pain is pain that starts suddenly and doesn't last long.

Dull pain is "a mild discomfort, often difficult to describe, that may be associated with some musculoskeletal injuries or some diseases of the visceral organs."[2]

A fifty-year-old has been in his or her body for fifty years; who best knows the fifty-year-old's body and the problems that have arrived: a stranger (such as a doctor) or the fifty-year-old?

Illness is considered poor health that results is sickness of the body or mind. The reasons people seek healthcare—and usually the way people measure their success with treatment.

Disease is defined as an abnormal condition of an organ, or system of an organism resulting from various causes, such as infection, inflammation, environmental factors, or genetic defect, and

---

[2] http://medical-dictionary.thefreedictionary.com/pain, disease, accessed June 20, 2017.

characterized by an identifiable group of signs, symptoms, or both. This is what needs to be 'cured,' especially if it's life-threatening.[3]

Many websites define illness as the feeling that comes with having a disease, such as pain, fatigue, weakness, discomfort, distress, or confusion, to name a few. These feelings are why people go to a doctor, thinking the doctor will have the answer. Then you have the word "disease," which is a different way of saying the same thing or nearly the same. I never liked that word, only because, I really didn't know the true meaning of it. For better clarity, a disease is a condition that affects different areas of the body, usually an organ or cells, and needs a cure to get rid of it. An "illness" is something people develop, such as a cold or pain that comes with some illnesses. Both are unhealthy conditions and needs to be addresses.

> *"And Jesus went about all Galilee, teaching in their synagogues, preaching the gospel of the kingdom, and healing all kinds of sickness and all kinds of disease among the people."*.[4]

---

[3] http://www.thefreedictionary.com/illness & http://www.thefreedictionary.com/disease/ Copyright © 2003-2017 Farlex, Inc
[4] Matthew 4:23 / (NIV via biblehub.com)

CHAPTER 2
First-Aid Kit

• • •

It is always a good idea to have a first-aid-kit available, you never know when one would come in handy. Putting a kit together yourself can aid in familiarizing yourself with certain products that really work or don't work. You can decide to incorporate some natural remedies as well, or make a separate kit. Make a kit for home use, or make one for storing in your vehicle. It could be a fun little project for the whole family. There are several sites on the Internet that you can get ideas from, or that provides ideas in putting together a more natural-remedy first-aid-kits, to just how to go about making them. I designed one by incorporating some essential oils and things I found to be health beneficial from just my cupboard. I found a military duffle bag to store it in for easy access. Some people get creative and use things like fishing tackle boxes and metal lunch boxes. The chart below is a useful guide to what can be used in putting in a first-aid kit.[5]

First-Aid Kit Item List	
Adhesive bandages	Bulb syringe
Liquid bandages	Dosage spoons
Thieves oil/sanitizer	Scissors

---

[5] http://www.home-storage-solutions-101.com/first-aid-kit-contents.html./ "Printable First Aid Kit Contents List," accessed June 20, 2017

Sterile gauze	Tweezers
Cold compress	Fine needle
DermaMed natural alternative to topical cortisone	Clove/birch oil for pain
Oatmeal alternative to Calamine lotion	Tylenol
Rubbing alcohol	Antacids
Hydrogen peroxide	Peppermint oil/nausea
Wash cloth/soap	Flaxseed oil/ginger root for anti-diarrhea
Eye wash solution	Oral electrolytes
Sterile saline solution	Rosemary essential oil alternative for mild laxative
Sunscreen	Antihistamines/Basil oil
Aloe Vera/Sunburn	Eucalyptus oil for bath for cold/flu
Cotton balls	Honey or Thieves for Cough
Cotton swabs	Prescription medicines
Disposable gloves	Cinnamon oil
Ace bandages	Thermometer

⁶God created heaven and the earth, and through His spirit, He gave the earth light and all the living things He made for His greatest creation, man. All that He made was good, for He blessed

each living thing. God made man in His own image, both male and female. He gave souls to both, and on the seventh day, God saw all that He had created was good, so He ended His work.

God also created a garden called Eden, and in the middle of that garden stood two trees, the "tree of life" and the "tree of knowledge of good and evil." He gave only one command or task, and it was never to eat from the tree of knowledge of good and evil. Everything was good until one day, the devil entered Eden and worked his evil, persuading Adam and Eve to disobey God. Instead of being grateful for all that God had given them—life, freedom, happiness, love, and goodness—Adam and Eve chose to trust evil over all the goodness they had. I believe that God gave man one simple task: to obey His will. God does good things for everyone out of love, and He wants nothing but joy and happiness for us. We choose to make bad decisions that cause bad results, and consequences come with bad decisions.

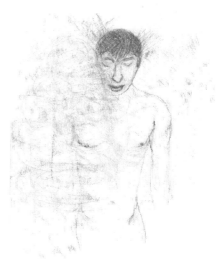

Figure 1 Sandy H. Durham God's Creation (Hidden Code Studios) 2017

> *Since choices often result in eternally significant consequences, we must choose in line with God's principles…It's possible to gain the whole world and lose your soul. There is much more in life than the outward and material. We must base our choices on God's Word, not on the assumptions of our culture. Those principles encompass the whole Bible and take a lifetime to learn thoroughly.*[7]

---

[7] "Lesson 28: Choices, Consequences (Genesis 13:5–18)," Bible.org, accessed June 20, 2017, https://bible.org/seriespage/lesson-28-choices-consequences-genesis-135-18.

Reading the Bible can give us a clearer understanding of God and how He works. The bible is the place you go to and find answers. Most of us believe that God created our bodies to heal naturally from illness and disease, since He did say that He created us in His image. (In my opinion, people get illnesses or diseases from the bad choices they have made or the environment they are in, it is free will, right? One can choose to make better choices, a bad choice/decision can have negative consequences. Take your time to make good choices/decisions, ask questions, turn to Gods word.

God forgives for all of our mistakes; we just need to ask Him for forgiveness. And even though we make bad choices in life, and illness results from it, I believe God built us in a way that if we can identify what we did that got us to that state, and if caught early enough the sickness/illness can be reversed. We can allow our bodies to heal naturally without all of the harmful prescription drugs that doctors prescribe. Prescription drugs have been known to do more harm than good. Most prescription drugs have more side effects that can cause health risks or even death, than it does doing good to treat the symptom.

As I look at my life before, I've found that the items I once used to aid in the management of my normal household cleaning, I realized it could be harmful to my family in the long-term. There was not one product we had that was not chemically made as far as ingredients. I started eliminating products one by one to some more healthier kinds. It was everything from haircare, makeup, toothcare, laundry products, foods, and outdoor yard products, I was so shocked. The supply of things that is available in our country I believe is far from God's original design.

For the word of the LORD is right and true; He is faithful in all He does. (Palms 33:4, New International Version, NIV)

As the years fly by, I am seeing our health-care system deteriorate because of federal involvement. A system flooded by health-care practitioners that leave us with no hope and no real answers to a lot of illness and disease issues. In my opinion, our health-care system is corrupted by federal bureaucracy and regulations that go nowhere but put us in early graves. I firmly believe that it will get worse before it gets better. Statistically, all types of illness and disease are on the rise. In my experience, most of the doctors I saw, had no desire to get to the cause of any illness, disease, or ailment I was going through. Why would they want me or anyone well? Conspiracy theorists say, that some doctors are motivated by profit, instead of the prospect of having healthier patients. They partner with the pharmaceutical companies to receive kickbacks and to keep everyone sick. They make more money when people are sick and not so much on the well visits or physical exams. On my journey to true healing, I asked questions and observed some true-life situations and journaled them. Also, when I saw the doctors and asked questions of things I knew through research, it seemed like they were angry at me for knowing stuff. But why?

Father God continue to give me the knowledge I need to understand my body, and how you designed it. As we all move through life, and we grow older, help us to unlock the essential information we need to know for our health, so that we can pass the knowledge on to others and to those that seek the truth. In Jesus, I pray, Amen!

CHAPTER 3
Observations

• • •

A TWENTY-SIX-YEAR OLD WOMAN SUFFERED many symptoms and some slight pain for a while. She went to several doctors, and none got to the bottom of her ailment; the doctors only treated her with prescription drugs. It wasn't until months later when she was hospitalized that she found out that she had leukemia, lymphoma, bone cancer, and stomach tumors. The discovery was made late in the game due to the bureaucracy of the health industry, and she ended up with massive and unbearable pain. The hospital gave her morphine that didn't provide the relief she needed. The leukemia had spread to her bones. Now the woman's fate was in the hands of the hospital and the medical bills are costing her and her family millions of dollars in unnecessary prescription drugs and treatment that in my opinion is just masking the root problem.

My mom told me the story of how my great-grandmother, Sarah, died. Sarah was remembered as a beautiful woman with no health issues until she was in her late fifties, she had been treated for gallbladder problems. Over time, her pains got worse, so the doctor decided to remove her gallbladder. When they opened her up, they realized that the source of her pain wasn't her gallbladder at all; it was cancer in her gut. She died at age sixty-two of stomach cancer. The doctor had misdiagnosed her.

Another story concerns a friend of my husband. This man had gone to the emergency room complaining of chest pains. Supposedly, he'd had a couple of heart attacks that he didn't know he was having. After some tests were performed, the doctors did surgery on him and found that one artery was completely blocked. The surgeon decided to put two stents in. After the man got out of surgery, he was taken to intensive care unit because his heart was only at 35 percent when it should have been at 50 percent. My gut feeling is that this should have been a red flag. It would have made me think that some other blockage was going on! Instead of checking for more blockages, the doctors only did what was necessary at that time, getting the heart pumping at a certain capacity. They would go back later if something else came up. What? Why wouldn't they do everything in one surgery instead of operating again later?

I learned that after my mom had her C-section during my twin and I's arrival, the OB/GYN doctor that preformed the C-section put her organs back in the wrong places. which later on caused a mass to build, then in turn caused her to have a total hysterectomy. I don't know about you but that sounds fishy to me.

I ask myself daily, are doctors really are that uncaring, clueless, and disconnected to patient care? Isn't that the reason they wanted to work in health care in the first place—to solve and correct illness? God put doctors in that field for a reason, right?

Another friend was also having heart trouble. He had fallen at work, and emergency medical technicians were called to take him to the hospital. But when he got there, the medical staff only monitored him and then released him. He later had a stroke that paralyzed one side of his body. If they had done more tests that day at the hospital, he probably wouldn't have had a stroke. The doctors at the hospital, in my opinion, didn't do the necessary tests to prevent the stroke from happening.

A different friend had been in and out of the hospital with an out-of-control potassium-level issue. Come to find out, other prescribed drugs she was taking were interfering with her potassium levels. It had caused her potassium level to get dangerously low, which could have potentially caused her heart to stop. I read that taking certain medications, can cause your methyl groups to get out of balance. With all of these issues, but what frustrated me the most, was that she was not asking necessary questions that should be asked. She was taking the medication she was given without asking what it was treating. I had told her to start asking questions before accepting treatment. Not all medications work for everyone. Sadly, my friend is no longer with us. In my opinion, the medications had life-threatening results. Rest in peace, my friend.

From these observations, I found that no one person asked the doctors any necessary questions, while they were in the hospital. I asked several friends who have been hospitalized, what kind of illness they were admitted with. None knew the details, but each person accepted treatment without knowing exactly what the medication was for. Asking a lot of questions is vital to healing properly.

Illness can be used by God to strengthen spiritual life:

And He said unto me, my grace is sufficient for thee: for my strength is made perfect in weakness. Most gladly therefore will I rather glory in my infirmities, that the power of Christ may rest upon me. (KJV)[8]

---

8 2 Corinthians 12:9 (KJV via Christianministries.org)

CHAPTER 4
My Backstory

• • •

My story begins a couple of years ago, when I first developed slight inflammation under my eyes. It started to concern me as it had not improved after a few weeks. I was starting to get irritated by the inflammation that was not only making my face puffy, but also making me look very aged. So, it was not long before I found myself addressing the problem of inflammation with my general practitioner. She examined me and thought it was only a severe case of indoor/outdoor allergies. She treated me with a steroid shot (Toradol, 60 mg), and the inflammation went away within a few days. A few weeks later, I assumed that the steroid had worn off as I then had developed a strange rash on my chest. I went back to my doctor, and she didn't think the rash was severe enough to worry about. Another week or so went by, and I noticed a new rash on the inside of my left upper arm one morning. It looked as though it was under the skin. The doctor wasn't familiar with this type of rash, so she referred me to a rheumatologist. My physician thought that the specialist would have more knowledge of this type of rash, and that he would be able to recommend the right blood tests. I told her that I didn't really want to be passed around from doctor to doctor, because I thought that as a general practitioner, she could do any kind of test, any other physicians could do. In the meantime, I already knew that I was allergic to certain molds and dust, from the testing I had done some time ago. My pastor had told me about some mold he found in his home that caused sickness, so he bought me an in-home air test kit to test the house we lived in at the time for mold. I tested the air-conditioning ducts, and the test read positive for some types of mold.

    I remember reading a story about Suzanne Somers becoming severely ill after she had been exposed to it. Prior to doing the mold test, I had considered another possible reason for what I was experiencing. I had remembered that I had taken a long course of antibiotics to control a recurring urinary tract infection (UTI). I did some research on the side effects that that particular medication could cause. During my research, I also found that some people had similar symptoms similar to those that I was experiencing. After I collected my findings, I talked to my physician about it. She assured me that there was no relationship between the antibiotics and the rashes that were showing up. She offered to do an autoimmune blood test to rule out illnesses such as lupus and arthritis. Incidentally, doctors don't usually tell people about the possible drugs that can trigger the onset of an autoimmune illness. In the meantime, my doctor continued to treat me with another dose of steroids to help with the inflammation. After a few weeks, she reviewed the test. It was negative, aside from showing a high antinuclear antibody (ANA), which just tells the doctor that inflammation is present in the body. She told me that with a high ANA, it had to be some type of autoimmune problem. At that point, not feeling confident with the outcome diagnosis, I wanted to continue with more blood testing. But all the tests I did came back normal. The doctor recommended that I consult with the rheumatologist. I was skeptical, but willing. I scheduled an appointment, and a few weeks later, my husband took time off from work to go with me. When we met with the rheumatologist, I gave him my thoughts on what it could be, I said to him, that I believed it had to do with the Nitrofurantoin medication I had taken for a UTI. He didn't think so, because he follows the half-life of medications. He then ran some blood tests, to rule out many of the things that my physician had initially considered. He literally gave me a thumb-up gesture, saying that he was leaning toward a diagnosis of dermatomyositis. When the blood work came back negative, he looked surprised, and only offered to give me a steroid shot to help with the inflammation, and then he suggested that I see a dermatologist, he said, she could do a biopsy of the rash to understand what it was. So, once again frustrated,

I was passed on to another specialist. I was still skeptical but willing to seek another opinion. I made an appointment with a well-known and highly recommended doctor of dermatology. My husband went with me one afternoon, and when we arrived and saw the doctor's glamorous lobby, we had an inclination that the visit was going to be very expensive. It was the biggest dermatology office I have ever seen. My husband and I sat in the lobby for a good twenty minutes before the assistant called my name. After spending some time in the examining room, the doctor finally came in. We thought she was somewhat arrogant; she displayed her diplomas and certifications all over the patient room. She talked to me for a while, I also mentioned to her that the rash might be a reaction to the UTI medication I had taken. She did not agree, stating that that drug would have been flushed out of my body by then. She recommended preforming a biopsy of the rash to see whether she could pinpoint the type of rash it was. She biopsied two areas, and in a few weeks, the biopsy report came back with a diagnosis of spongiotic dermatitis.

Spongiotic dermatitis, is a type of an acute eczema effecting the skin. It's usually an extremely itchy rash that appears on the arms and legs and in some people with severe cases can cause permanent scaring.

In my case, my symptoms of itching were mainly on my hands, and legs and somewhat of my feet. I was reading an article and it is said that certain environmental triggers can cause an onset. We are constantly exposed to tons of man-made substances in the environment that cause illness. Allergist say that certain regions of the US are more effected by allergies. Texas is one of the regions that effects tons of people to have severe allergies. I have heard that things like perfumes, colognes, cleaners, abnormal hormone levels to even stress, can trigger certain allergies to be present and also could be a catalyst for the onset of an autoimmune disease. Triggers are different from person to person, when you do identify something you could be allergic to, write it down in your journal for things to avoid. I started with food allergy and sensitivities, by following an elimination diet and documenting everything.

So, as the story continues, now really feeling let down and frustrated, the dermatologist did nothing to find the root cause or fix the problem, other than prescribe a topical steroid cream, I paid a lot of money for a biopsy and a prescription. Time continued to pass by, I didn't know what group of doctors to try next. Being so let down and really surprised by the fact none of the doctors I saw, didn't have any answers and didn't do anything to further investigate what I was dealing with. By then, the itchiness all over my body got more severe, but mainly on my hands, for several months. The inflammation is still present today in my hands and feet, knees, and ankles. Recently, itchy rashes appeared above my left knee and on my right shin. After my diagnosis, I continued to do my own research, very confused as to why no specialist so far had an answer for me. They all seemed to be confident that it was an autoimmune disorder and did not look to the patient for any perspective. I felt like they were only interested in getting me in and out of the office, yet to appease me in their mind, they were glad to provide another prescription or shot but, no real answers.

None of the doctors mentioned that autoimmune is an underlying condition, and not a root cause.

From my view, I am still leaning on that it is an allergic reaction to something, or a trigger of some sort. Regardless, I read that autoimmune illnesses can start in the gut and is reversible. So, I started a twenty-one-day juice regimen to see where it would take me. It was very hard to stick to at first, especially when my family and friends were eating things that smelled too good to pass up, but I was strong and kept with it. At the end of the juice regimen, I had lost ten pounds. I was excited; I felt energetic, clothes fit me better, and my face looked clear and vibrant. I am glad that I tried juicing, I had nothing but positive results. I would recommend juicing to anyone.

As my story continues, through word of mouth, I found a place called the Environmental Health Center located in Dallas, Texas, which is known for conducting extensive test and therapies. I was thrilled, as this place seemed very promising. I continue to use their services as my journey continues daily.

With that being said, through extensive research I started in my late twenties, I had diagnosed myself with Friedreich's ataxia (FA). I found the symptoms and said "that's got to be it!" The research gave me the clues that I needed, and Friedreich's ataxia matched my symptoms. Eventually, it was confirmed with a blood test. Who diagnosed me was a doctor of neurology at the University of Texas Southwestern Medical Center. Still at this time this disease was not well known to the medical world, due to the limited amount of cases, or at least that is what I was told. In any event, my findings were shown to be accurate. Currently, there is not a cure for Friedreich's Ataxia, yet. This condition has to do with an iron overload in the mitochondria and a synapse disconnect, in which case needed signals cannot be sent to the brain. Ultimately, I learned that no one in my family on either side has suffered this type of disease. My thoughts of me having FA, and not being in my family history, leads me to believe that it may have been a trigger by something that I was exposed to in my teenage years, or when my mom was pregnant with me and my identical twin sister. The strangest thing, a Godsend really, we seem to have split this disease, and because of that, we don't have many of the effects that most people with FA suffer with. My twin also lives in the Midwest, so she is around different environmental irritants than I am exposed to here in Texas, maybe that is why we have different repeats from each other. Researching the disease, I learned that the frataxin gene on chromosome 9 is expanded with nonsense information known as a triple repeat. This extra DNA interferes with the normal production of frataxin, thereby impairing iron transport. Normally, there are between ten to twenty-one repeats of the frataxin gene. We are excited as more new news continues to come out around FA, and as it does we will meet and learn more. My only concern is the possibility of researchers developing drugs for FA will be a synthetic one, which I have read most drugs are developed with this element, which in the long run causes side effects and bringing back illness.

While I feel as though we would all love to have a quick fix when we fall ill, our bodies are a lot more complicated than that. I continued doing research to get to the bottom of my itchy rash problem, and through word of mouth, I came across a middle-aged woman who had beaten colon cancer through diet. She had also opened a holistic wellness center here in Texas. She mentioned that she had attended a health program at the Optimum Health Institute (OHI) in San Diego, California, where she had learned about healing through, all-natural, holistic practices. The program focuses on the physical, mental, emotional, and spiritual well-being. I visited her facility, and right away she did a thermography exam with the Diacom machine to analyze other parts of the body. I learned some interesting things how these two device types give out information with specific attributes that provided some type of solution options. On a different visit, I tried out another machine called Riffe, it uses different frequencies that targets different organs and tissues in the body. This type of therapy requires a series of uses, some people notice a difference of how they feel after only a few sessions.

> *Father God, thank you for each and every day you give us on Earth. Please forgive us for the way this world has become. Father, open our eyes to the way things should be. Guide us and direct us. Heal our bodies and cleanse our world. In Jesus's mighty name I pray. Amen!*

I finally visited the Environmental Health Center of Dallas, and met with the facility's founding physician. After talking to me and examining me, the doctor wanted to check how my immune system was functioning, so he ordered a T and B lymphocyte subset profile. This test analyzes the fighter cells which are the T cells in the body. The test came back normal, so the doctor, wanting to investigate further, so he then recommended preforming a cell-mediated immunity test (CMI). This test analyzes the performance of the T & B cells and gives an understanding of the level at which the immune system is working. The results showed that my immune system is not performing at the level it should be and is not as responsive as it should be.

The doctor got a good understanding of how my immune system was working, so he recommended that I undergo a blood draw for the treatment needed to fix my immune problem. The treatment, called Autogenous Lymphocytic Factor (ALF), is made from the patient's own blood. It is a mixture of effector substances that may be released from the patient's own stimulated healthy T lymphocytes. As a biological response modifier, ALF is created under strictly controlled conditions. It is composed of over two hundred proteins. When immune cells are placed in cell culture, the weak die and the healthy become robust. First, the blood is drawn and sent to the lab. Within two to six weeks, it is sent back, and the doctor administers the first dose to determine the strength needed to build up the immune system. This type of treatment can be given for up to a year, as determined by the doctor, and then repeated tests are done to determine whether the ALF is working.

The doctor also recommended that I undergo some skin testing to identify any allergies to things like chemicals, molds, and foods and thus either confirm or rule out any allergy to mold or any chemical exposure that could have caused the persistent rashes. On this visit, I decided to try the intravenous therapy, which is meant to supply the necessary nutrients depleted from the body. Individuals wanting a rapid detoxifier also use this type of therapy. Doing this type of therapy will boost the immune system function, and replenish any depleted nutrient throughout the body. After I completed this therapy, I felt a welcome burst of energy. The Environmental Health Center offers so many different kinds of therapies. I am confident that with continued tests, I will get closer to finding a solution for my condition.[9]

Thank you, Father God, for giving me the strength and direction to find the right people who will discover the root cause of my illness. Thank you for the peace and hope I feel in knowing that the answer is coming and that I will soon be on my way to feeling better. Amen!

---

9 Generic patient information/EHCD/flyer

CHAPTER 5
Root Cause

• • •

IF YOU REALLY THINK ABOUT the term "root cause," makes total sense, to me. When a plant gets sick, the first thing to examine is the root system to find the root that is causing the plant to be sick.

Another analogy is to imagine how the fictional detective Sherlock Holmes used differential diagnosis to solve crimes. By observing many clues and how they are related to the crime, Holmes determines who the criminal was. Medical schools supposedly teach a systematic technique[10], for identifying patients' diseases. A medical condition must be identified, before it can be treated. Differential diagnosis, [11]is a form of scientific reasoning. The way I understand it, in most scenarios, a medical doctor's first step is evaluating the patient's symptoms, and reviewing his or her personal and family history. Then, the physician does a quick differential

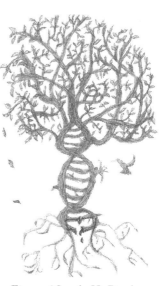

Figure 2 Sandy H. Durham Root Cause, "Tree of Life" (Hidden Code Studios) 2017

---
10 umuc.ed/using systematic technique/online writing
11 https://en.wikipedia.org/wiki/Differential_diagnosis

diagnosis of what may be causing the ailment. Next, the doctor could perform tests to eliminate the possibility of a certain illnesses, until the most likely one shows up positive. Once the illness has been identified through the process of elimination, the doctor then can prescribe a therapy. Usually, a drug is given to the patient as part of treatment. If the patient doesn't show improvement in a given time frame, the diagnosis is then reevaluated, and a different treatment continues. Doctors today have so many patients they don't have time to get to the root causes of their patients' ailments, and they don't disclose any of the harmful side effects of the medications they are prescribing. Ultimately, prescription drugs can cause additional problems. Especially, when a person takes multiple medications the more complicated it becomes molecularly.

When we want to find the root cause of disease, we have to understand how to tackle it. Logically, we know that when we see a plant that has a sickly look about it and is always losing its leaves or flowers, we know we can't just cut off the bad leaf to make it all better and healthy again. You need to go to the root of the plant to fix the problem. Supposedly, a similar process is used in the medical world to deal with physical illness and disease, yeah right, lol. We come across imbalances in our bodies all the time. Treating only the visual symptoms is not enough! We must dig deeper, discover the root cause, and treat the issue in order to bring about complete healing. Depending on how deep an illness/sickness is, healing can take a while. It may take months or years, and in some cases, a lifetime. Just remember, healing is a journey. Everything has purpose and reason, pray God shows you the purpose.

A band aid has its purpose; it is used to protect and keep wounds clean during the healing process. We don't need a bandage all the time. Always have faith and patience and believe that the answer will be found. I came across a blog in Today's World, Rick Piña writes, "Faith without patience produces people who start off good, but burn out over time. Patience without faith produces people who constantly suffer, but have no power to change their situation."[12] We have to have both faith and patience. These two combined will enable us to inherit the promises.

Rejoice in hope, be patient in tribulation, be constant in prayer. (Rom. 12:12)

Through whom we have gained access by faith into this grace in which we now stand. And we boast in the hope of the glory of God. Not only so, but we also glory in our sufferings, because we know that suffering produces perseverance, character, and hope. (Romans 5:24 NIV)

---

12 Rick Piña, *Today's World*, accessed June 20, 2017, http://todaysword.org/

CHAPTER 6
Building an Action Plan

• • •

MOST PEOPLE DON'T KNOW HOW to differentiate between the two types of illness. It is very important to understand the differences between a virus and a bacterial illness. Remember that a virus has to take its course. Going to the doctor to get an antibiotic is unnecessary because antibiotics only work on bacterial illnesses and some bacterial causing viral infections. So, if you have a simple cold or flu bug, taking antibiotics will not make it go away. *It has to take its course.*

In general, people have gotten too complacent. Example being, when they see their practitioner, they automatically expect to leave with a prescription. Most of the time, doctors do not hesitate in writing antibiotic prescriptions, whenever a patient asks for one. They make more money when writing prescriptions. My suggestion, is to avoid the temptation of asking for a prescription if it is not really needed. Instead, ask what you can do to feel better without taking medications or how to take a more natural approach.

If you must have the magic pill remedy, always take your prescriptions as directed. Always follow the prescribed instructions and read about the adverse side effects. Add all of the information to your health journal to better track reactions. Never skip any doses, even if you start feeling better. Stopping any prescribed medication prematurely, can cause the illness to come back, and the result will require more antibiotics, and possibly a higher dosage that might not work as well. Always discard any remaining antibiotics properly; never flush them down the toilet. You should never consider taking someone else's prescriptions, because sharing antibiotics, never ends positively. You are unique; one medication doesn't work the same for everyone. I always wondered why medications are developed for everybody, and not made for the individual by a person's body weight and DNA. I know some pharmacies do compounding[13]

Remember when you were little, and your mother always told you to wash up before dinner? Some mothers—like mine—were always warning us not to touch anything with our hands—to use a foot, or an elbow instead, momma said, that doing this would protect us from bad bacteria.

To help protect against the spread of bad bacteria, you only need to wash your hands with soap and water then dry them well. If you are in the hospital or visiting someone in the hospital, wash and dry your hands before and after visiting. Some say that using antibacterial cleansers is too extreme, and that using soap and water is best. So, if this is true, why are hospitals today, using hand sanitizers located by every patient room door. Looking at some third-world countries, I believe that those people are stronger than most of us in the United States of America because they are exposed to the environment they live in and medications are not overprescribed. Therefore, their bodies are better able to fight off bad viruses or diseases. Have you ever heard of someone's grandpa saying to roll around in the dirt? Supposedly, it will keep you from getting sick. I believe if we weren't so overly medicated we could handle our natural environment.

---

13 Pharmaceutical compounding/ is the creation of a particular pharmaceutical product to fit the unique need of a patient

CHAPTER 7
Questions Confirmed
• • •

IF YOU HAVE DONE YOUR research on your DNA regarding certain markers that call out certain disease and illness, and discovered that autoimmune diseases are not primarily in your DNA, the cause is likely from a different source. In some cases, antibiotics or environmental factors can trigger autoimmune illnesses. If you did a DNA analysis from places like 23andme and you see that you have some markers of illness that could arise. They tell you just because it shows a marker(s) doesn't mean you will get the disease or illness. If you haven't done a DNA analysis, 23andme is a reputable company, and they make it so easy for everyone.

Autoimmune disease such as rheumatic fever or streptococcal infection can follow infections that your body has had. When I did a Diacom test it showed that strep was still in my tissues. Interesting fact, some bacterial infections has been linked to bring on certain autoimmune illnesses. When your body becomes overloaded with certain nutrients this also has been linked to autoimmune disease. I read that too much iodine in your body for example, can contribute to the onset of autoimmune thyroid disease. In most cases, environmental triggers can bring about an onset of autoimmune disease, but the medical community hasn't pinpointed what. That's why it's helpful to keep a heath journal describing any changes that take place with anything you change such as, treatments and any additions or subtractions to your diet or environment. Journaling is a great way to find or pinpoint any strange occurrences, and can be a starting point in researching illness or anything that arises. I wish I would have started a journal before I got ill, this would have helped me in the discovery phase of my illness.

Our bodies are always being invaded by bacteria, viruses, and other foreign pathogens. Our bodies are normally strong enough to fight off these invaders, and no harm occurs. Sometimes intruders or pathogenic bugs are very difficult to get rid of. Certain individuals who have weakened immune systems have difficulty fighting off the foreign pathogens they are exposed to such as, *Borrelia burgdorferi*[14], *Babesia microti*[15], *and Candida albicans*[16]. If you suspect that you have been exposed to one of these pathogens, get tested. These diseases created by these pathogens can cause your immune system to be hyperactive and cross-react with normal tissues in the body. People who have been exposed to many of these factors show symptoms of autoimmune illnesses and produce autoimmune markers in blood tests.

If you are suffering, be patient; God is already working on the solution. Don't sit, do your research. God gave us authority to move forward. Rebuke the enemy from taking over your patience, and have faith in Him. Remember that everything is in His hands and that He is working for good. In John 10:10 (New International Version,

---

14 a bacterial species causing Lyme disease in humans and borreliosis in dogs, cattle, and possibly horses. The vector transmitting this spirochete to humans is the ixodid tick, *Ixodes dammini*. http://medical-dictionary.thefreedictionary.com/Borrelia+burgdorferi, Segen's Medical Dictionary. © 2012 Farlex, Inc. All rights reserved.

15 The babesiosis agent, an intraerythrocytic protozoan parasite endemic in rodents, Peromyscus spp and Microtus spp, and which is transmitted to humans via a tick, Ixodes dammini. Segen's Medical Dictionary. © 2012 Farlex, Inc. All rights reserved.

16 a common budding yeast; a microscopic fungal organism normally present in the mucous membranes of the mouth, intestinal tract, and vagina of healthy people. McGraw-Hill Concise Dictionary of Modern Medicine. © 2002 by The McGraw-Hill Companies, Inc.

NIV), the thief comes only to steal, kill, and destroy. [17] Sickness steals, kills, and destroys. Jesus said that we might have and enjoy life and health in abundance—to the fullest, till it overflows.

Father God, we thank You always for the life You give us. We continue to seek Your guidance and grace. Put us on the right path that will lead us to the answers we seek. We know You are the greatest physician. You heal, protect, and love. Bind us with Your loving hands. We ask for continued strength and faith. Forgive us if we stray and do not hold strong in our faith that You are always working out those things we worry about. We love You with every fiber of our bodies. We ask this in Your son Jesus's name. Amen!

---

[17] John 10:10 New International Version (NIV), The thief comes only to steal and kill and destroy; I have come that they may have life, and have it to the full.

CHAPTER 8
Healthy Heart

• • •

I THINK IT IS IMPORTANT to understand how our hearts function it is a crucial organ to understand to stay healthy. Without the heart, we would not live. Understand how your heart functions, and then write in your journal about how you feel.

A normal, healthy heart pushes the blood though the blood vessels, arteries, veins, and capillaries that comprise the circulatory system, carrying throughout the body the necessary oxygen and nutrients that each organ needs. An electrical system controls the heart. When the heart walls contract, blood is pumped into the circulatory system. Inlet and outlet valves in the heart chambers ensure that blood flows in the right direction. The blood in our bodies also carries carbon dioxide so that we can breathe in oxygen and expel carbon dioxide.

A normal, healthy heart is usually as big as your fist and located in the center of your chest, just under the rib cage, between the right and left lung. An average adult heart rate is around seventy to seventy-five beats per minute that pumps is about five liters of blood per minute. Children's heart rates average eighty to ninety beats per minute, depending on their age. An adult's average "resting" heart rate is around sixty to one hundred beats per minute. The heart rate should be around 220 beats per minute minus your age, when you are doing any kind of physical fitness activity.

There is a mathematical equation that cardiologist use to measure a person's heart function. The power of the heart can be calculated by multiplying the pressure by the flow rate. An average person has six liters of blood that circulates every minute, making the flow rate 10^{-4} m³/s (cubic meters per second). The pressure of the heart is about 10^4 pascals, making the heart's power about one watt. This is the power of a typical human heart, but it's different for everyone.[18]

Looking at the diagram, the heart has four chambers. The upper two chambers are the atria, and the lower two are the ventricles. The chambers are separated by a wall of tissue called the septum. Blood is pumped through the chambers, aided by four heart valves. The valves open and close to let the blood flow in only one direction.

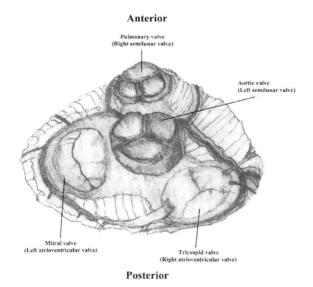

Figure 3 Sandy H. Durham "Heart valve" (Hidden Code Studios 2017

---

18 http://hypertextbook.com/facts/2003/IradaMuslumova.shtml

The four heart valves are:

1. The tricuspid valve, located between the right atrium and the right ventricle.
2. The pulmonary (pulmonic) valve, is located between the right ventricle and the pulmonary artery.
3. The mitral valve, is located between the left atrium and left ventricle.
4. The aortic valve, is located between the left ventricle and the aorta.

Each valve has a set of "flaps" or leaflets or cusps. The mitral valve normally has two flaps; the others have three.

From The body To The heart
The dark bluish blood, is low in oxygen, the blood flows back to the heart after circulating through the body. It returns to the heart through veins and enters the right atrium. This chamber empties blood through the tricuspid valve into the right ventricle.

From the heart to the lungs
The right ventricle pumps the blood under low pressure through the pulmonary valve into the pulmonary artery. From there the blood goes to the lungs, where it gets fresh oxygen.

After the blood, has been re-oxygenated it is bright red. Then the blood returns to the left heart through the pulmonary veins to the left atrium. From there, it passes through the mitral valve and enters the left ventricle.

The left ventricle pumps the red oxygen-rich blood out through the aortic valve into the aorta. The aorta takes blood to the body's general circulation. The blood pressure in the left ventricle is the same as the pressure measured in the arm.

Everything is as God made it; not as it appears to us. We have the world so much in our hearts, are so taken up with thoughts and cares of worldly things that we have neither time nor spirit to see God's hand in them. The world has not only gained possession of the heart, but has formed thoughts against the beauty of God's works. We mistake if we think we were born for ourselves; no, it is our business to do good in this life, which is short and uncertain; we have but little time to be doing good, therefore we should redeem time. Satisfaction with Divine Providence, is having faith that all things work together for good to them that love him. God doeth all, that men should fear before him. The world, as it has been, is, and will be. There has no change befallen us, nor has any temptation by it taken us, but such as is common to men. (Matthew Henry's commentary on Eccles. 3:11–15)

Keeping the Beat

It is important to manage your heart rate during any kind of physical exercise. Training or exercising is an important time to chart your heart rate. Take into consideration this average heart-rate chart; it will give you a guideline on a good target heart rate when exercising. Then write it in your journal.

Age	Target HR	Average Maximum HR,
20	100–170 beats per minute	200 beats per minute
30	95–162 beats per minute	190 beats per minute
35	93–157 beats per minute	185 beats per minute

40	90–153 beats per minute	180 beats per minute
45	88–149 beats per minute	175 beats per minute
50	85–145 beats per minute	165 beats per minute
60	80–136 beats per minute	160 beats per minute
65	78–132 beats per minute	155 beats per minute
70	75–128 beats per minute	150 beats per minute

Important Note: Some high-blood-pressure medications can give a lower maximum heart rate. always consult with a professional before starting any workout regimen—especially if you have any heart or health conditions.

According to scripture the time He walked the Earth Jesus healed the spirit of people first by laying hands on them, and through His spirit they were healed and their bodies were restored. He also gave His disciples like Peter this same gift of healing the spirit of the people then restoring their bodies.

He gave us all this same gift, we can through Jesus Christ and with the Holy Spirit lay hands on people requiring spiritual healing. God calls people into different roles and occupations so that their gifts and strengths can be used to care for others, and bring glory to Him. Each gift is meant to be used in His name for His glory. Being a physician is a gift that should be used to glorify Jesus by helping others. It's clear that many doctors today have blinders on and have no real purpose other than to seek monetary perks. In Romans, the apostle Paul states that we have different gifts, according to the grace given to us. Furthermore, God placed upon the hearts of some to become a doctor in the world to heal people, sadly their focus is only on the body and not the spirit. So, this is the problem, and must be fixed. Physicians need to look more holistically at the person like Jesus Christ did, first fix the spirit and second restore the physical body. Until this optic is refocused physicians will continue to misdiagnose, because without the spirit the body in not complete.

There are so many theories regarding doctors in biblical times. I've read that in that time people had limited means of diagnosing and treating illness. In fact, illness was said to be due to sin or an enemy's curse. In the Old Testament, there are very few references to physicians found and for good reason. Jesus used the physician references to aid in educating the Pharisees to understand the link between both the physical and spiritual person. Ancient Greek refer to physicians being trained by the Egyptians. During the time of Jesus, Rome was said to be an important medical center where physicians practiced. Julius Caesar granted citizenship to physicians who would practice in Rome. The Greeks knew a physician's job in the first century was to heal people.

Ultimately, God through his son, Jesus Christ, is the true healer and is demonstrated by Mark and Luke who tell the story of a woman who had sought the help of physicians but had not been healed (Mark 5:24–34 and Luke 8:42–48). From the story told, it is clear that healing from a physician did not occur, is was only with her pure faith and by touching the fringe of Jesus garment was she immediately healed.

While Jesus walked the earth, he was the physician, yet his focus was not on the physical body but instead the spirit within which is the root cause to the pains we feel and the sicknesses we experience. To be clear, God needs no middleman. Jesus preformed miraculous healings when He was on Earth, but there was always one requirement; faith, the person seeking to be healed had to believe and have unshakable faith in God, His father.

O Lord, by these things men live, and in all these is the life of my spirit. Oh, restore me to health and make me live!

If you are someone that is suffering from health issues, God has a plan and a real purpose for you, embrace your sickness remember God did not heal Paul from the thorn he had in his side, God said to him, "My grace is sufficient for you, for my power is made perfect in weakness. Therefore, I will boast all the more gladly about my weaknesses, so that Christ's power may rest on me." 2 Corinthians 12:9

Trust in the Lord with all your heart, and do not lean on your own understanding. In all your ways acknowledge him, and he will make straight your paths.
Proverbs 3:5-6 New International Version (NIV)

When Jesus was here on Earth and someone went to Him for healing, Jesus, healed the person directly and personally. God blesses each of us with different gifts and occupations. If a man's gift is prophesying, let him use it in proportion to his faith. If it is serving, let him serve; if it is teaching, let him teach; if it is encouraging, let him encourage; if it is contributing to the needs of others, let him give generously; if it is leadership, let him govern diligently; if it is showing mercy, let him do it cheerfully (Romans 12:6-8). [19]Be proactive, don't procrastinate, make a change for the betterment of you and your health. Take ownership now of your health and spiritual well-being. You will find by making this change, it is rewarding and brings a longer, healthier life. Your health is your responsibility, not something that should be delegated to others. We can uncover most ailments and disease through research. Always keep a positive attitude, because attitude plays a huge role in restoring health. Be positive be proactive, research, journal, keep faith, trust, and believe that God's healing is coming. start the choice now!

---

19 Romans 12:6–8 (NLV via Biblehub.com/

You know your body better than anyone else does, and prescription drugs are not always the answer to health problems. Of course, if it is a matter of life or death, taking a prescription drug might be the answer, but prayer definitely is the first true medicine. He will guide you by prayer which path you should take. Keep your ears and eyes wide open, a message could come through someone else or signs. Because you have so little faith. Truly I tell you, if you have faith as small as a mustard seed, you can say to this mountain, "Move from here to there," and it will move.[20] Nothing will be impossible for you.

To understand the complexity of how prescription drugs, work in a person's life, take this example: An eighty-two-year-old man was diagnosed with first Parkinson's, and was treated for the disease for a few years. Then he was re-diagnosed with MLS, which is much worse than just Parkinson's and in order to 'manage' these diseases he has to take more than twenty-two different medications and the matrix of reactions is so complex. All these medications are doing nothing more than keeping the symptoms suppressed, yet they are not resolving anything only masking the real problem. Why would the 'educated' medical industry 'mask' the problem instead of searching for the real or 'root cause' problem to formulate a very real solution.

It's evident that prescription drugs are on the rise. And with the more drugs people are taking, bigger drug cabinets are needed. I pray for all those people suffering with illness and only getting the band-aid job for a solution. I do not understand why most people do not care about the harm medications are causing. It seems as though we have given up on seeing what the body really can do on its own. God gave us so many things for survival, we need to use our brains and try those things that God put on the earth first. You have nothing to lose. Just research it!

---

20 Mathew 17:20 (NLV via biblehub.com).

People living in the United States have become slaves to the perceived quick fix and adapted to what they think is free handouts. In reality, though, nothing is free. Everything in life is work, and we must at least try. We can do anything we put our minds to and accomplish positive results. Even if we fail, we can learn by our failures and come back stronger. With our illnesses, if we want to turn them around, we can do it. I should have followed my own advice I wouldn't have wasted valuable time and money on all of the medical appointments I have gone to, and hoping that one of the doctors would find answers and give a real solution to my illness. Have you experienced this? Everything happens for a reason, right?

Shouldn't doctors be getting to the root cause before prescribing? In my experience, doctors I saw were quick to prescribe prescription drugs without knowing what the root of the illness was. Why? I have never been willing to pay big bucks for a bandage. In an article, I found titled, "Pharmaceutical Company Corruption and the Moral Crisis in Medicine," Sharon Batt writes, "Doctors are just masking the illnesses and ultimately causing additional problems." They are sending us down the path of a plethora of personal prescription drugs. Do you feel as though the health-care industry and government have fallen away from the spiritual walk with God and the true purpose of health-care? I am saddened to see that going to a doctor is not the answer most of the time. Doing my own research has been a rewarding and positive experience in the management of my health. We all need to learn more about certain sicknesses and how are bodies function so we can stop going to the doctor for every little thing. Learn the difference between viral and bacterial infections. See to it that no one takes you captive through philosophy and empty deception, according to the tradition of men, according to the elementary principles of the world, rather than according to Christ.[21]

---

21 Colossians 2:8 (NIV via biblehub.com)

CHAPTER 9
Bacteria and Virus

• • •

I MENTIONED EARLIER THAT IT is important to differentiate between bacteria and a virus, in doctor lingo it's either a viral or bacterial illnesses. There are many types of bacteria, both good and bad and can be found everywhere like in the air, soil, on your skin, or in and on your body. Bacteria adapts to and can handle extreme environments, either extreme cold or extreme heat. Most bacteria are no threat to people; other types cause sicknesses, such as strep throat, tuberculosis, or urinary tract infections.

Also, if you misuse and or overuse antibiotics, bacterial illnesses can develop, and can become resistant to treatment. I have dealt with many different types of bacteria in my lifetime, having had UTIs, strep throat, and bad bacterium on my thumbnail, to name a few. All of these illnesses required taking some sort of medication to get rid of them.

It's important that we keep a good balance of good bacteria or gut flora, for our system to function properly. There are three types of gut flora that plays a specific role in the human body;

1.) **Essential Flora**[22]: This is the good/friendly bacteria that is found in the gut. In healthy individuals, essential flora dominates and controls other types of less desirable microorganisms.

---
22 all the plants of a particular area or period of time, (Definition of "flora" from the Cambridge Academic Content Dictionary © Cambridge University Press)

When functioning normally, this type of flora is responsible for conducting numerous roles that keep the body healthy.

2.) **Opportunistic Flora:** This group of microbes is found in the gut in limited numbers, and are strictly controlled by the essential flora in a healthy person. This type of flora is capable of causing disease if the essential flora becomes compromised, and is unable to control the growth and numbers of opportunistic flora.

3.) **Transitional Flora:** These are various microorganisms that are introduced into the body through eating and drinking. When the essential flora is, healthy and functioning normally, this type of flora, will pass through the digestive track without causing harm. However, if the essential flora is damaged, this group of microbes can cause disease.[23] Most people (myself included) incorporate probiotics into their daily diet as they are good for a healthy gut.

When normal flora bacteria become too numerous, or gets disrupted by foreign pathogens, they then can cause infections like urinary tract infections and other infections in different areas of our body. Example of bacteria that causes illness;

Escherichia coli (commonly called E. coli) lives in the colon, aiding in the digestion of food and preparing for the elimination of waste from the body. It generates vitamin K that aids in blood clotting.

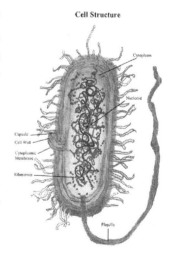

Figure 4 Sandy H. Durham "Bacteria" (Hidden Code Studios) 2017

---

23 https://www.sott.net/article/267668-The-Forgotten-Organ-Gut-flora-and-its-role-in-immune-function

Our immune system establishes mechanisms to stop, contain, or attack these pathogens should they enter the body. Bad bacteria can cause infection and illness by killing the cells they attack, or by releasing toxins. Antibiotic medications are most common in treating bacterial infections. Today, researchers have been studying the ends and outs of the gut flora, how the immune system functions, also how health and disease begins in the gut. Facts show, that 80-85 percent of the immune system resides in our guts (the second brain). In a healthy individual, the gut flora protects one against viruses, parasites, toxins, and undigested food particles, by forming a layer of gut flora that coats all of the digestive tract. This type of bacteria also controls the pH in our bodies, making it hard for microbes to survive; neutralizing toxins, controlling and eradicating harmful carcinogens that would cause cancer cell development and growth. This study has been helpful for doctors in choosing the right type of antibiotics for patients needing to treat bacterial illnesses.

Other advances in the study of molecular medicine, now have a better understanding of the function of bacteria, how it supportive in health and how it would cause illness. Viruses are different in size and shape from bacteria, and can only replicate on a living host. Viruses attack human cell's and can replicate very quickly by taking over the cell, and making the inside of the cell its home. Viruses can change the genetic material of the host cells normal makeup, then take over as a virus. Most viruses have to run its course, but some can be treated for its symptoms and spreading, while other viruses are very lethal. It's a good idea to keep track of how your immune system is functioning, because if your immune system is not fighting off viruses and other intruding pathogens, it would be difficult to get well, because of its ability to multiply. When a virus takes over a cell and multiplies, infection can set in making it more contagious. According to the medical community, there is no method that can provide our bodies the same level of defense against all viruses, only some of them.

However, we know that our bodies have the ability to heal by itself. When we are subjected to a virus, our body learns its DNA or RNA patterns, and if the body successfully defends itself against a virus, it can, and will defend itself again the next time it confronts that virus. It is so very important to recognize that the symptoms caused by viruses—such as fever, vomiting, and tiredness—are a result of the body's defense mechanisms kicking in, to eradicate the virus from the body. In many cases of cold and flu, the immune system destroys the infection, because it remembers the DNA or RNA patterns from another attack. I remember having measles as a child, and not only was I able to fend off this virus but now my body remembers its DNA or RNA pattern, so I will not have to fight it off again. This gives me life-long resistance to the measles virus. This past year, for the first time, I got a virus that attacked the larynx called laryngitis. Maybe when my immune system was low, my body became vulnerable to virus. Also, when my son played ice hockey years ago, I got a virus called Bell's palsy, which attacked the facial muscles and paralyzes them. When this happened, I ended up going to the ER, not knowing what it was I was dealing with. The doctor knew, and said that it had to take its course, so I had to deal with the drooling anytime I took a drink or brushed my teeth. It was so strange. If you get a virus, just remember that it usually has to take its course. Stay strong, ask a physician to do a test, to see what type of virus you are dealing with, and stay positive; it will get better soon.

Father God if we get a virus, help us to trust our body to function the way you designed it to perform. Give us the patience to see it through to the end. Thank you for sending your son Jesus to take on all our sins and give us a new life. Thank you Father for the individual purpose you give us, help us to understand what our purpose is so we can overcome, the things that we are meant to endure. I pray for healing for all, and long life in Jesus name Amen!

CHAPTER 10

Look Up in the Air! It's Superbug!

• • •

HAVE YOU HEARD OF THE term "superbug?" No it's not a super hero type of thing, it's a real epidemic that is happening all across the world? Superbugs begin when a bacterium enters the human body, and has become resistant against any medications we would take to heal or control from spreading. Some bacterium that become resistant to antibiotic medication; like Staph, Methicillin-resistant Staphylococcus aureus (MRSA), Escherichia coli (E. coli), and Carbapenem-resistant Enterobacteria (CRE) are amongst the known. The biggest places that are prone to superbugs, are hospitals, and health care facilities. America is the most overly medicated country in the world, and someday, there will be bacteria that our bodies will not be able to fight off, even with the strongest antibiotics available. The superbug will be resistant to the medications that we would need to save our lives, someday. This

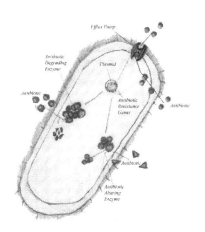

Figure 5 Sandy H. Durham "Super Bug" (Hidden Code Studios) 2017

scary theory is getting closer to becoming our reality. I ask myself (and you should too) what people would do if they could not get their prescriptions filled. What would happen if a catastrophic event occurred and prescription drugs were unavailable or unable to be manufactured? I can only imagine that millions of Americans could be faced with some really hard times. When we talk about superbugs, we have not even begun to understand the ramifications of all the medications we have been taking in our lifetime. I continue to worry for family members, as most continue to accept that prescription drugs are the answer; they are not seeing the bigger picture when it comes to the future and what superbugs will do to them. Physicians who always prescribe antibiotics to stop viruses and other things that just treat symptoms should know what they are causing. We have to change this behavior before it is too late.

When I had a thermography, and used the Diacom machine, it showed that many of the bacteria that can bring on illness were still in my body, including strep and staph. What I want to know is, if these bad bacteria are still in my body, why have my doctors not done something about it? My biggest concern is for infants and children, whose bodies are highly susceptible to bacterial infections. Parents should seriously take into consideration that their children are still developing, and they should take a more natural approach to their children's health by limiting their consumption of antibiotics. Superbugs are a more serious problem than most are aware of, particularly at places like hospitals, colleges, food processing plants, and nursing homes, just to name a few. Hospitals and any facilities that care for small children or the elderly should especially have a system in place for cleaning properly to minimize the possibility of outbreaks. There are reports that superbugs have taken the lives of people that are constantly taking antibiotics unnecessarily. Cancer is soon to be low on the list of problems, in the near future due to superbugs.

Speaking of the chemicals in medications that in turn cause a superbug scenario, we also need to realize those same types of chemicals is also in the foods we eat. For the people that are not worried about the processed foods they buy, these foods are becoming more dangerous to consumers to consume, because of the number of chemicals the food is processed with. With more animals and foods produced today, farmers are having to follow certain restrictions before sending their commodities to the markets. Molecularly speaking, people are eating meats that are processed with antibiotics and hormones that are then absorbed into their bodies. Not only are we being exposed to environmental challenges, now we are also limiting our own bodies' ability to properly fight off bacteria and virus, just by eating the food we buy and consume. God, help us get back to the ways you intended.

Father God protect our bodies from all the harmful drugs that man is subjecting us too. please forgive us, for falling short of your will. help us, to stay on track for anything you set for us to accomplish. Thank you again for our lives, and challenges we face, and for all the prayers you have already answered. I pray for our future, and that this world gets closer to you. in the name of Jesus, I pray, Amen!

CHAPTER 11
The Drug Effect

• • •

I HAVE HAD FOR SOME reason an almost measurable or rhythmic UTI occurrence, that at least twice a year I would get this type of bacterial infection. I remember the day I met with my OBGYN physician, and after dealing with this re-occurring infection, he recommended that I be on a long-term regiment of an antibiotic medication to aid in keeping the UTI at bay. I could say that while I was on the regiment, I did not have another UTI. On the flip side, from keeping the infection at bay, I could only call it the 'drug effect'. My feeling and thought was that this type of treatment or medication, was causing the reoccurrences? Why was the physician not looking into the root cause, before prescribing? This whole problem I have now, may be the trigger for the illness I am dealing with.

For years, I have seen commercials marketing new drugs on television. After a while my husband and I have made a game of counting the number of side effects to the medications being advertised. We had counted more than twenty-eight side effects with one drug. One can only ask, 'are the side effects better than the health problem they are masking. *Bottom line*: it seems obvious to me that, it is worse or even fatal taking the medication then actually dealing with the illness, what is up with that? I have read that people living in the United States of America, from adolescents to those over age fifty, are among the highest users of prescription drugs, and this is leading to drug abuse or death, according to studies. I believe that the illness I have, started with medications I took and with time the effects of taking them. I don't believe that physicians really follow the half-life, they are articulating. The physicians I was passed around to, didn't ask if I had previously had a steroid shot, but gave me one. Does this seem, right?

Dear friend, I pray that you may enjoy good health and that all may go well with you, even as your soul is getting along well[24]

---

24 3 John 1:2 (NLV via Biblehub.com)

CHAPTER 12
The Drug's Life

• • •

THIS CAME UP WHEN VISITING my physician. I asked my doctor about the amount of time a drug stays in your body. My physician mentioned the medical community follows the half-life of prescription drugs. To better understand the factors and effects of medications in the body, I needed to know how the body metabolizes drugs. Here is a baseline formula for half-life and clearance rate for almost any prescription drug:

$$t_{½} = \frac{\ln \cdot V_D}{CL}$$

With this formula, the variables are defined below for half-life, volume of distribution and clearance:

Half-life (t½): is the time required to decrease half the amount of drug in the body.
Volume of distribution (VD): of a drug represents the degree to which a drug is distributed in body tissue rather than the plasma.
Clearance (CL): is a pharmacokinetic measurement of the volume of plasma from which a substance is completely removed per unit time.

A person's metabolism can change the clearance rate from the bloodstream and affect the speed at which a drug is processed. In case you needed to be reminded, both the liver and kidneys are very important in this process.

The liver is a site of drug metabolism, and the kidneys are crucial in blood filtration and are one of the most important organs for unchanged drug/drug metabolites elimination.

Many factors can affect how long a drug lasts in a person's body, including age, sex, social factors, genetic factors, and diet.

So, we do not lose heart. Though our outer self is wasting away, our inner self is being renewed day by day. For this light momentary affliction is preparing for us an eternal weight of glory beyond all comparison, as we look not to the things that are seen but to the things that are unseen. For the things that are seen are transient, but the things that are unseen are eternal.[25]

---

25 2 Corinthians 4:16-18 (NIV via Bible.is,)

CHAPTER 13
Cells

• • •

GOD DESIGNED OUR BODIES VERY precise, unique, and very complex. Therefore, looking at the internal makeup, the different cells in the body perform different functions, each one essential to the overall health of the body. When I was researching my illness, I read that from the trillions of cells in the body,

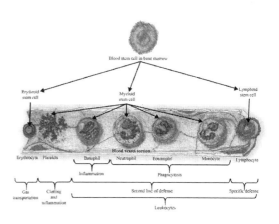

*Figure 6 Sandy H. Durham "Cells" *Hidden Code Studios) 2017*

the ones that play a role in the immune system, or that help balance hormones, could be playing a part in what I was going through. When it comes to the cells in the body, all of the trillions of them have specific jobs they perform. Most unite to build body parts such as organs, muscle, skin, and bone. Groups of different types of cells make up the organs in your body, such as your heart, liver, or lungs. Each organ has its own job to do as well, but all organs work together to maintain your body. Each cell in our bodies, are covered by membranes as barriers that protects each cell. The cells are grouped and organized into certain routine jobs types like; nerve, brain, and the red and white blood cells. Proper nutrients, and oxygen is necessary and is an important part of survival. Certain diseases can destroy cells, as is the case with Friedrich's ataxia. This may be why the disease progresses. I was diagnosed with FA through UT Southwestern, but most of the blood test I did recently, was done through the Environmental Health Center. You can get most blood test done through specialists or ask your doctor about blood test options. Understanding what test might be good to check, and can give a better understanding what cells do what function, and can provide an idea which blood test you would start with or consider testing. Whatever test you do definitely journal your results, this will help you to identify changes.

The T and B cell test, is not a normal test that a general practitioner will perform. The T and B cells make up the immune system. The test is a simple blood draw, and it can take up to fourteen days to get the results back. When your results do come back, have your doctor explain what is a normal reading and what is not. It is important to understand, as these cells work together in keeping your immune system strong. All of these cells are subsets of the lymphocytes, or white blood cells. Below are definitions I found to be helpful:

- **CD3**: found on T helper (Th) and T cytotoxic (Tc) lymphocytes; associated with signal transduction.
- **CD4**: found on T helper lymphocytes; an adhesion molecule that binds to class II MHC molecules.
- **CD8**: found on T cytotoxic and variably on NK lymphocytes; an adhesion molecule that binds to class I MHC molecules.
- **CD19**: a type I, transmembrane protein found on all B cells and B-cell precursors, and some follicular [26]dendritic

---

26 http://medical-dictionary.thefreedictionary.com

cells, that acts as an accessory molecule for B-cell signal transduction.

The white blood cells are known as the fighter cells as they attack foreign bodies. Among these are the CD3 cells—the mainframe or master control cells—and the CD4 cells, which are known as helper cells because they activate the T cells. The T cells control immune system function and are responsible for protecting and healing damaged organ systems. You also have CD8 cells, known as the suppressor cells, and CD19 cells, known as the natural killer cells. The T and B test tells how many fighter cells (or soldier cells) a person has. Usually, the doctor will combine the T and B test with a delayed immune test (DIT), which tells you how well your fighter-cells are functioning. Over time, we all get exposed to a wide array of environmental irritants or toxins that can affect our T and B cells. When your body becomes infected with a foreign germ, the T and B cells will respond: they quickly multiply, creating an army of identical cells to fight the infection.

My T and B test was normal, so my next test was a cell-mediated immunity (CMI) test. This is an invaluable assessment of the immune response of the T lymphocytes that sometimes become weakened by allergies or environmental substances. This test is administered with eight different base pathogenic serums connected to small syringes that are pushed into your forearm for twenty seconds. Yes, this test is very painful, but it is well worth the short-term pain you have to endure. The technician performing the test will draw a ticktacktoe marking that separates each pathogen that is also numbered. You then, wait forty-eight hours to see how your body responds and then return to the office so that your doctor can analyze the results.

In my health research, I wanted to know more about the mitochondria sense my ataxia has to do with it, this is what I found. The mitochondria are described as the power plants of the cells.

"Mitochondria is a membrane bound cellular structure and is found in most of the eukaryotic cells. Also, referred as organelles, supposedly they generate most of the energy of the cell in the form of adenosine triphosphate (ATP) and it is used as a source of chemical energy. The mitochondria are also involved in other cellular activities like signaling, cellular differentiation, cell senescence and also control of cell cycle and cell growth. Mitochondria also affects human health, like mitochondrial disorder and cardiac dysfunction, and they also play an important role in the aging process". Friedreich's ataxia, the disease I have, has to do with the mitochondria in the ninth chromosome.

"Although mitochondria are present in every cell, they are found in high concentrations in the muscle cells that require more energy. Though the primary function of mitochondria is to produce energy, they also play an important role in the metabolism and synthesis of certain other substances in the body."[27]

Another cell that is important in health that you may have heard of, is the Cytokine. This cell is a generic term for non-antibody proteins. The cytokine is released by one cell population on contact with a specific antigen, which acts as intercellular mediators, as in the generation of an immune response.[28]

The dendritic cells are another type of cell that has a big role in the immune function. This cell is a type of antigen-presenting cell (APC) that can be found in the adaptive immune system, also known as the

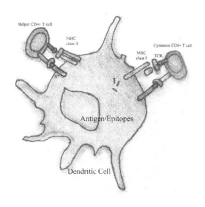

Figure 7 Sandy H. Durham "Dendritic cell" (Hidden Code Studios) 2017

---

27 http://www.buzzle.com/articles/mitochondria-structure-and-functions.html
28 http://medical-dictionary.thefreedictionary.com/cytokine

gatekeepers. The main function of dendritic cells is to present antigens to the CD4 T cells. These cells are therefore sometimes referred to as 'professional' APCs (antigen preforming cells). Dendritic cells also contribute to the function of B cells and help maintain their immune memory. Dendritic producing cytokines and other factors that promote B cell activation and differentiation. Dendritic cells are found in tissue that has contact with the outside environment such as the over the skin, and in the linings of the nose, lungs, stomach and intestines. Immature forms are also found in the blood. Once activated, dendritic cells move to the lymph tissue to interact with T cells and B cells and help shape the adaptive immune response.

The lymphatic system is also a defense system for the body. It filters out organisms that cause disease, produces white blood cells, and generates disease-fighting antibodies. It also distributes fluids and nutrients in the body and drains excess fluids and protein so that tissues do not swell. [29]The lymphatic system is made up of a network of vessels that help circulate body fluids. These vessels carry excess fluid away from the spaces between tissues and organs and return it to the bloodstream.

I praise you, for I am fearfully and wonderfully made. Wonderful are your works; my soul knows it very well. - Psalm 139:14 (NIV)[30]

---

29 https://www.news-medical.net/health/What-are-Dendritic-Cells.aspx
30 Psalm 139:14 (NIV via Biblehub.com,)

CHAPTER 14
Deoxyribonucleic Acid (DNA)

• • •

OUR GENETIC MAKEUP IS so complex and unique for everyone, I am an identical twin and scientist say identical twins share the same DNA, but we are so different in many ways. The strangest thing is both my twin and I have FA. While doing my research, I found that no one in my family has had nor experienced any like symptoms of FA. This is interesting as both parents would need to be a carrier of the genetic mutation to pass along to my sister and I. Furthermore, the genetic marker goes much deeper than only my parents, it would need to have been found somewhere in their genealogy. This is where I feel like an anomaly, as both my sister and I had a very late onset of FA. We were not diagnosed until we were in our late twenties and do not carry the holistic symptoms of FA. Neither my twin or I have the heart arrhythmia nor the spinal curvature or even speech impediments which are predominate characteristic of FA. In fact, it was four years later after being diagnosed that the FA had progressed enough that I needed to use a walking aid in order to get around. As discussed earlier in the section titled 'My Back Story' where FA has been discovered in the 9th chromosome as it relates to the mitochondria, this is the purpose for exploring, in depth the DNA. DNA is another important factor in how each individual is linked to a disease and how he or she handles the disease. There are many resources that allow for a genomic sequencing of your particular DNA. I suggest you take the time and precaution to understand your own DNA. Forms of DNA testing provides a wide array of information that can aid in understanding yourself and your reaction to medications and environmental elements based on several kinds of markers.

Knowing or finding a marker in your DNA does not indicated that you will get that disease or disorder, but you could if your life style is not managed. Knowing which diseases or disorders you are susceptible to, can help in deciding what type of lifestyle is right for you.

Technology has advanced so rapidly these last fifty years that the research available can and is overwhelming. The sheer amount of data available from a specific patient alone is challenging; it is clear to me why physicians are unable to effectively reach a root cause for their patients. Most physicians are not equipped to leverage or adopt such technologies as IBM's Watson[31] or other artificial intelligence like technologies that will ultimately advance healthcare more effectively. Physicians should have the information to specifically and especially know their patients' overall wellness. A key to breaking this barrier is to better understand some of the simpler elements of individual's health such as lifestyle along with their diet and nutrition. A company out of California called 23andMe which does DNA testing that delves deeply into a person's health and also provides ancestry information.

Another component of the DNA as it interferes with the immune system. Is DNA methylation and is part of epigenetics this field of study might be a positive turning point for cures. During my

---

[31] Watson is a question answering computer system capable of answering questions posed in natural language, developed in IBM's DeepQA project by a research team led by principal investigator David Ferrucci https://www.ibm.com/watson/health/

research, and reading further about DNA methylation seems like it could be a link to how FA works as far as gene expression. I feel like it is important to further understand methylation to see if it could be the key component and a critical part to healing of illness.

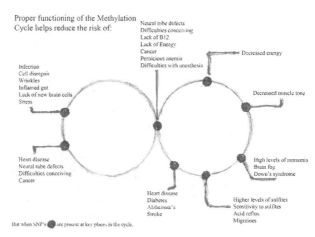

Figure 8 Sandy H. Durham "Methylation" (Hidden Code Studios) 2017

I have read that if you have a shortage of methyl groups, or your methylation cycle is interrupted, you could get sick. "Methylation is the process of taking a single carbon and three hydrogens, known as a methyl group, and applying it to countless critical functions in your body such as: thinking, repairing DNA, turning on and off genes, fighting infections, and getting rid of environmental toxins. [32]"Research has clearly linked impaired methylation with autoimmune conditions." [33]In fact, "given the critical role of DNA methylation in gene expression and cell differentiation, it seems obvious that errors in methylation could give rise to a number of devastating consequences, including various diseases. Medical scientists are currently studying the connections between methylation abnormalities and diseases such as cancer, lupus, muscular dystrophy, and a range of birth defects that appear to be caused by defective imprinting mechanisms."[34]

---

32 https://wordpress.com/read/blogs/75548436/posts/20763
33 https://existwell.com/2017/07/18/finding-balance-with-methylation-synergy-supreme/
34 https://mindbodyfitness.us/2017/05/15/methylation/

CHAPTER 15
Immune System

• • •

I NEEDED TO BETTER UNDERSTAND how the immune system works since my immune system got compromised somehow. Our immune system is our body's protection or defense system, and it is always at work. As I discussed previously and knowing that my immune system was compromised I needed to learn more and in great detail of how the immune system should function. As I learned more it allowed me to clearly relate the relationships between the actions and reactions within my body. Below is a clear description of the elements to consider as you research your own immune function.

The immune system has two main parts, the innate/natural immunity system and the adaptive/acquired immunity system. The innate/natural immunity system a general defense against pathogens, it is also called the nonspecific immune system. Mine was in both the first and second line, specifically in the skin from what I could best describe as netting pattern (looked like a birthmark) and inflammation of the joints (hands, knees and ankles). It works mostly at the level of immune cells called either the scavenger cells or killer cells. These cells mostly fight against bacterial infections.

The adaptive/acquired immunity system has specialized cells, like the antibodies that target very specific pathogens that the body has already had contact with. By constantly adapting and learning the body, these cells can also fight against bacteria or viruses that change over time. After reviewing my own T cell and B Cells information I found it was normal. My next test was a cell-mediated immunity (CMI) test which was off. As mentioned in the chapter 'Cells' knowing this information is key to your continued research for your own health. These immune systems do not work independently of each other. They complement each other in any reaction to a pathogen or harmful substance, and are closely connected. These two immune systems are complex in design, and they work constantly to fend off foreign invaders such as bacteria, microbes, toxins, and pathogens such as viruses and parasites.

CHAPTER 16
Immune Response System
• • •

NEXT ARE SOME CONSIDERATIONS WHEN understanding the characteristics of the immune response system

The immune response follows two paths, one using cytotoxic T cells and one using B cells. Normal cells of the body that become infected can also digest some of the pathogens and display antigen fragments on their cell surfaces. The body makes millions of different types of cytotoxic T cells each type is able to recognize a particular antigen. The cytotoxic T cells that are capable of recognizing the antigen displayed on the surface of infected cells bind to the infected cells and produce chemicals that kill the infected cell. Death of the infected cells results in destruction of the pathogen. These cells also come in millions of different types, each able to recognize a particular antigen. When B cells become activated by T helper cells they differentiate into plasma cells. These plasma cells become antibody producing factories, flooding the blood stream with antibodies that combined to the antigen involved in this infection. Antibodies bind to the antigens on the surfaces of the pathogens marking them for destruction by macrophages. Some of the B cells do not turn into antibody factories but instead become memory B cells that they survived for several decades. Because of these memory, B cells the secondary immune response to a future infection by the same pathogen is swifter and stronger. This powerful secondary immune response is what gives your body immunity to some diseases, after you have had it once or after you have been vaccinated.

There are three types of response systems in the immune system: the anatomic response, the inflammatory response, and the immune response. The anatomic response is the branch of the peripheral nervous system that regulates the function of your internal organs, like the heart and stomach. It also controls your smooth and cardiac muscles and your glands. I had dealt with one of the immune responses which was the inflammatory responses our second line of defense.

The inflammatory response begins when injured tissue cells release chemical signals that activate the endothelial cells of nearby capillaries. Within the capillaries adhesion molecules called selectins are displayed on the activated on the endothelial cells. These adhesion molecules attract neutrophils slow them down and cause the neutrophils to roll along the endothelium. As the neutrophils roll along the endothelium, they encounter chemicals that activate integrins, which are adhesion receptors on their surfaces. These integrins then tightly attach to adhesion receptor molecules on the endothelial cells. This causes the neutrophils to stick to the endothelium and stop rolling. This accumulation of neutrophils along the walls of the capillary is called margination. The inflammatory mediators released by the injured tissue bring about changes in the body that cause

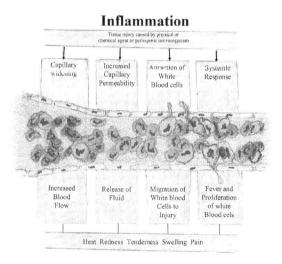

Figure 9 Sandy H. Durham "Inflammation" (Hidden Code Studios) 2017

mast cells to de-granulate and release histamine. Histamine causes vasodilation, and an opening of the junctions between the endothelial cells allowing fluid and leukocytes to leave the capillary and enter the infected tissue. The neutrophils now undergo dramatic changes in shape, and squeeze through the endothelial wall into the interstitial tissue and fluid. This process is called extravasation. The neutrophils followed by other types of phagocytes are attracted to the damaged site by packed substances released by bacteria and tissue breakdown products. They ingest and destroy invading bacteria.

When the inflammatory response fails, the immune response is activated and goes to work—typically, when a pathogen enters the body. Macrophages [35] that encounter the pathogen ingest, process and display the antigen fragments on their cell surfaces. Macrophages with antigen fragments displayed on their surfaces are called antigen presenting cell. An Antigen presenting macrophage interacts with a T-helper cell that can recognize the same antigen. During the interaction, the macrophage releases a chemical alarm system called Interleukin-1, which stimulates the T-helper cell to secrete interleukin two interleukin-2. Interlukin-2 causes the proliferation of certain cytotoxic T cells and B cells.

The sympathetic nervous system gets you ready for activity (the fight-or-flight response) and the other undoes what the other did. It is called the parasympathetic nervous system, and it is responsible for maintaining your body and conserving energy. Together they create feelings of stress, fear, relaxation, defiance, courage, panic, and peace, to name a few. Their nerve fibers originate in different parts of the body. The nerves of the sympathetic nervous system originate between your thoracic and lumbar vertebrae, which is called the thoracic lumbar area.

---

[35] a phagocytic tissue cell of the immune system that may be fixed or freely motile, is derived from a monocyte, functions in the destruction of foreign antigens (such as bacteria and viruses), and serves as an antigen-presenting cell, "Macrophage." *Merriam-Webster.com*. Merriam-Webster, n.d. Web. 9 Oct. 2017.

The nerves of the parasympathetic nervous system sprout from the base of your brain and from the craniosacral area superior to your tailbone. Both parts require two neurons in order to work, and these neurons meet in ganglia, clusters of neuron cell bodies that house millions of synapses. The neurons themselves have slightly different forms, namely the length of their axons. The neuron before the ganglion is called the preganglionic cell. The neuron coming out is the postganglionic cell, which is much shorter in length. The structure of each of these systems is related to its function.

Cells and molecules of the host gather at the sites where they are needed in order to eliminate the offending agents. Looking at our body's immune system, there are three lines of defense against foreign pathogens: the physical and chemical barriers (innate immunity), nonspecific resistance (innate immunity), and the specific resistance (acquired immunity).

The 1st line response of the Innate/Natural immunity (non-specific response) includes the physical barriers such as our skin, which is the largest organ. Our skin (epidermis) periodically sheds cells, removing any microbes. Our mucus membranes produce mucus, which traps microbes. Hairs in the nose filter air that carries microbes, dust, or pollutants. Cilia, which lines the upper respiratory tract, also traps and propels inhaled debris that enter the throat. When we urinate, the urine flushes out microbes in the urethra. Additionally, a part of the physical barrier or mechanical removal that is responsible for causing vomiting and defecation does this by expelling microorganisms out of the body.

When the 1st line of defense becomes compromised, the second line of defense goes to battle and destroys foreign pathogens in a generalized manor. The phagocytic cells fight by ingesting microbes that get into the body tissues. Macrophages are the white blood cells that leave the bloodstream and enter body tissues, patrolling for microbes. Fever is another nonspecific resistance in innate immunity. Every cell in our bodies have a specific job to do, always fighting to keep one well.

The 2nd line response of the Innate/Natural immunity (nonspecific response) includes chemical barriers. Lysozyme, which is an enzyme produced in our tears, perspiration, and saliva, goes to work killing off bacteria by breaking down cell walls and secreting its own antibiotic. The gastric juices in our stomachs destroy bacteria and toxins because it is acidic. Our skin produces acids that can inhibit bacterial growth, and it has a protective film called sebum (unsaturated fatty acids). From every cell and fiber in our bodies is always working to destroy what shouldn't be in/on our body. That's amazing!

The way I understand it, inflammation is the body's nonspecific response when injury or illness occurs. Inflammation is defined as a complex response of vascularized tissues to infections and damaged tissues. The inflammatory response can be provoked by physical, chemical, and biologic agents, including mechanical trauma, exposure to excessive amounts of sunlight, x-rays and radioactive materials, corrosive chemicals, extremes of heat and cold, or by infectious agents such as bacteria, viruses, and other pathogenic microorganisms. Although these infectious agents can produce inflammation, infection and inflammation are not synonymous. The classic signs of inflammation are heat, redness, swelling, pain, and loss of function. These are manifestations of the physiologic changes that occur during the inflammatory process.

The 3rd line response of the adaptive/acquired immunity system (specific response) called the specific resistance or acquired immunity. It is an adaptive immune response. Specific resistance relies on antigens which are proteins found in the foreign microbe serving as the stimulus that activate the immune response. The term antigen comes from antibody generating substance. If you want to find out more details around the immune system and how it functions, research (functions of the immune system).

Father God help us to understand our inflictions I know we all are not healed because your grace is sufficient for us but whatever we become inflicted with help us to stay strong in faith and keep you in the forefront Thank you for my life and your mercy in Jesus name Amen!

CHAPTER 17
Autoimmunity & Causes

• • •

I HEARD A LOT OF diseases derive from the gut so we need to better understand the gut, and how it functions. The gut is described as a hollow muscular tube made of layers of cells that are divided into two sections; the small and large intestines. The small intestines are divided into three parts 1ˢᵗ the Duodenum[36], Jejunum[37], and Ileum.[38] By the time food reaches your small intestine, it has already been broken up and mashed into liquid by your stomach acids. Each day, your small intestine receives between one and three gallons (or six to twelve liters) of this liquid. The small intestine carries out most of the digestive process, absorbing almost all of the nutrients you get from foods into your bloodstream. The walls of the small intestine make digestive juices, or enzymes, that work together with enzymes from the liver and pancreas to do this.

Looking at the small intestine as a pipe, it seems hard to believe that an organ so narrow could do such a big job. However, looks can be deceiving. The absorptive surface area of the small intestine is

---

36 The short section is the part of the small intestine that takes in semi-digested food from your stomach through the pylorus, and continues the digestion process.
37 The middle section of the small intestine carries food through rapidly, with wave-like muscle contractions, towards the ileum.
38 This last section is the longest part of your small intestine. The ileum is where most of the nutrients from your food are absorbed before emptying into the large intestine.

actually almost 2,700 square feet—the size of a tennis court! How is this possible? The small intestine has three features which allow it to have such a huge absorptive surface area packed into a relatively small space, the Mucosal folds,[39] Villi,[40] and Microvilli.[41]

Although the small intestine is narrower than the large intestine, it is actually the longest section of your digestive tube, measuring about twenty-two feet on average, or three-and-a-half times the length of your body. Your large intestine is about five feet long. The large intestine is much broader than the small intestine and takes a much straighter path through your belly, or abdomen. Its job is to absorb water and salts from the material that has not been digested as food, and get rid of any waste products left over. By the time food mixed with digestive juices reaches your large intestine, most digestion and absorption has already taken place. What's left is mainly fiber (plant matter which takes a long time to digest), dead cells shed from the lining of your intestines, salt, bile pigments (which give this digested matter its color), and water. In the large intestine, bacteria feed on this mixture. These helpful bacteria produce valuable vitamins that are absorbed into your blood, and they also help digest fiber. The large intestine is made up of Cecum[42], Colon[43]. The colon consists of four parts; Ascending: Using muscle contractions, this

---

39 The inner surface of the small intestine is not flat, but thrown into circular folds. This not only increases the surface area, but helps regulate the flow of digested food through your intestine.

40 The fold's form numerous tiny projections which stick out into the open space inside your small intestine (or lumen), and are covered with cells that help absorb nutrients from the food that passes through.

41 The cells on the villi are packed full of tiny hair like structures called microvilli. This helps increase the surface of each individual cell, meaning that each cell can absorb more nutrients.

42 This first section of your large intestine looks like a pouch, about two inches long. It takes in digested liquid from the ileum and passes it on to the colon.

43 This is the major section of the large intestine; you may have heard people talk about the colon on its own. The colon is also the principal place for water reabsorption, and absorbs salts when needed.

part of the colon pushes any undigested debris up from the cecum to a location just under the right lower end of the liver. Transverse: food moves through this second portion of the colon, across your front (or anterior) abdominal wall, traveling from left to right just under your stomach. Descending: the third portion of colon pushes its contents from just near the spleen, down to the lower left side of your abdomen. Sigmoid: The final S-shaped length of the colon, curves inward among the coils of your small intestine, then empties into the rectum.

The rectum, is the final section of digestive tract, it measures from 1 to 1.6 inches. Leftover waste collects there, expanding the rectum, until you go to the bathroom. At that time, it is ready to be emptied through your anus.

CHAPTER 18
Molecular-Level Autoimmunity

• • •

AUTOIMMUNE DISEASE CAN STRIKE ANYONE. There are over millions of cases in the United States alone. There are around 140 cases of diseases that have been classified as autoimmune disease, and is steadily rising every year especially among women. Although doctors don't say that autoimmune disease is reversible, it is in most cases. Remember, I talked in a previous section about choices we make like what you eat, how much you exercise, how you live your life, and what you're exposed to every day, from the agricultural chemicals, industrial toxins, and pollution, all can have an effect on your health. Since our bodies are made of millions of cells, and when the body gets exposed to antigens, similar molecules found in some disease-causing microorganisms, have been identified on specific cells and tissues in the body.

Molecular mimicry is defined as the theoretical possibility that similarities in frequencies between foreign and self-peptides are sufficient to result in the cross-activation of autoreactive T or B cells, by pathogen-derived peptides. Molecular mimicry is one explanation for autoimmune diseases. After contracting infection with a microorganism whose surface contains antigens similar to those found in the body, the immune system may respond inappropriately by trying to damage these cells that have similar surface antigens in otherwise healthy joints, blood vessels, or other organs. Molecular mimicry is structural, functional and have immunological similarities shared between macromolecules found on infectious pathogens in host tissues. Infection may induce autoimmune responses which attack and destroy body tissues or organs. Normally, the body is tolerant to self-antigens which are present in individual tissues. In autoimmune disease, Tolerance involves non-self-discrimination, which is the ability of the normal immune system to recognize and respond to foreign antigens, but not self-antigens. Autoimmunity is evoked when this tolerance to self-antigen is broken. Molecular mimicry of a self-antigen by an infectious pathogen, such as bacteria and viruses, may trigger autoimmune disease due to a cross-reactive immune response against the infection. Cross-reactive antigen–antibody and T cell–antigen reactions are used to identify the mimicking macromolecules on the pathogen and in tissues or organs.

CHAPTER 19
Causes of Autoimmune Disease

• • •

THE CAUSE OF AUTOIMMUNE ILLNESSES is unknown, but people talk about triggers such as certain bacteria, viruses, drugs, chemicals, and environmental pollutants that can bring on autoimmune disease. I hear that most autoimmune conditions derive from the gut, so possibly we can reverse them by eating healthier, like feeding our bodies lots of organic green veggies, to reboot our guts and systems. Eating foods that the body doesn't agree with or has a sensitivity to, can cause the immune system to be out of balance, and this leads to the immune cells acting as if our own tissues are foreign. If you are someone that has sensitivities to certain foods, but you are not sure which foods they are, I suggest tackling it the way I did by using process of elimination, to pinpoint the foods that are in question. Also, finding what makes you irritable or stressed is also plays an important role to good health. Your emotions can also affect your health as well; this is called oxidative stress. Getting plenty of rest is just as important to health, and not oversleeping. Another cause of autoimmune disease could be an overgrowth of small bacteria in the small and large intestine. It is helpful to ingest good bacteria such as acidophilus to keep the gut flora in check. Foreign opportunistic pathogen [44]cause the immune system to

---

[44] an organism that exists harmlessly as part of the normal human body environment and does not become a health threat until the body's immune system fails.

become overactive, leading to chronic inflammation. When this happens, the immune system becomes confused about what is foreign in the body and what is not, leading to various autoimmune diseases. Symptoms that you could experience getting this type of condition are fatigue, gastric pain or other abdominal issues. To be sure you can have certain doctors check for overactive Immune.

A person's hormones are a factor in autoimmune illness. If the hormones are not in balance—for example an increased estrogen/progesterone ratio in women or decreased cortisol production from long-term stress could lead to a multitude of ailments such as rheumatoid arthritis, lupus, and Hashimoto's thyroiditis.

A leaky gut can cause an increased intestinal permeability[45], which can lead to autoimmune illness. I personally did the twenty-one-day juice diet, thinking that if I had leaky gut it would fix the gut. Sometimes, a person can be exposed to heavy metals that can cause our body to be too toxic. If this sounds like you, it might be a good idea to do some testing. Look into labs such as Spectra Laboratories that do micronutrient testing. I talk about micronutrients in the next chapter of this manuscript.

---

45 Gastrointestinal tract dysfunction caused by antibiotics, toxins, poor diet, parasites or infections, leading to increased intestinal wall permeability and absorption of toxins, bacteria, fungi, parasites, etc.; LGS may be linked to allergy and autoimmunity. Another term leaky gut syndrome

CHAPTER 20
Micronutrients

• • •

EVERYTHING PERTAINING TO THE HEALTH and wellness of our bodies is around making sure we are providing proper elements to insure we give our bodies what it needs to do its job better. One more of these things is proper nutrients. Our bodies need the proper nutrients in order to be in balance and to function properly. These nutrients are broken down into two categories, micronutrients and macronutrients. The meaning of micronutrients is in the name—micro meaning very small or microscopic. Even though your body needs only very small amounts of micronutrients, being deficient in a micronutrient can lead to huge health problems. Most of the vitamins and minerals that are difficult to obtain through a normal diet are micronutrients, including vitamins A, C, D, E, K, B6, B12, thiamin, riboflavin, niacin, folate, biotin, and pantothenic acid; and sodium, potassium, calcium, magnesium, phosphorus, manganese, zinc, copper, selenium, iron, iodine, chromium, molybdenum, chloride, and cholesterol.

Some of the food we eat also supplies our bodies with micronutrients. It is an important to get these nutrients into our bodies to provide the energy we need, growth, and all the functions that our body produces. The macronutrients are categorized as carbohydrates (sugar), four calories per gram; lipids (fats), nine calories per gram; and proteins, four calories per gram. Macronutrients make up the calories we take in. It is very important to take in the right number of macronutrients to be healthy. Some of the macronutrients need and what it is good for is listed below.

- *Manganese* promotes bone formation and energy production, and helps your body metabolize the macronutrients, protein, carbohydrate and fat.
- *Magnesium* helps your heart maintain its normal rhythm. It helps your body convert glucose (blood sugar) into energy, and it is necessary for the metabolizing of the micronutrients calcium and vitamin C.
- *Iron* helps your body produce red blood cells and lymphocytes.
- *Iodine* helps your thyroid gland develop and function. It helps your body to metabolize fats, and promotes energy production and growth.
- *Chloride* helps regulate water and electrolytes within your cells, as well as helping to maintain appropriate cellular pH.

Micronutrient testing is not typically provided by a normal practitioner, but most health insurances will cover this type of testing. Check with your insurance company first. Micronutrient tests screen for deficiencies in vitamins, minerals, amino acids, antioxidants, spectrox (antioxidant function), carbohydrate metabolism, fatty acids, and metabolites. Many places do micronutrient testing. Just search the Internet for micronutrient test labs in your area. Recording the micronutrient test and any dietary changes that is suggested through any micronutrient tests is another good use for your health journal. I did an extensive micronutrient test through my chiropractic and wellness physician. When I got the results back, I was able to purchase the micronutrients that I was deficient in through the same physician.

CHAPTER 21
Journaling

• • •

A JOURNAL OR DIARY OF your choosing, is the best way to keep track of your health changes through your life. You can design a journal yourself or use the many apps or templates you can find on the internet. Journaling will help you to provide a trackable history of events, which will aid in connecting the dots as you move to finding and or establishing the root causes of any health issues. The more information you add, the better. It can assist you in the future or as health issues arrive. I made my own health journal it is very detailed. Your physician keeps a medical history of all his or her patients, including you. Journaling is your own personal health history document. You can bring it with you when you visit your physician if a health issue does arise, so that he or she can see what you've done in the past regarding your health.

Keeping a journal for some might seem like a lot of work to manage, but in the end well worth it. Stick with it because you never know when something might arise, and you realize that the effort you put in it became a necessity. Doing a journal might take some time to populate, eventually you will see the positive results of all the things you wrote regarding your health by following through. Trust me, results will happen and when those results do show up, you can take pride in knowing that, with the help of your journal, you were able to pinpoint some root causes to some illnesses that arise. Here are the facts some facts on health journaling.

In life, you can pinpoint Patterns: If you are someone that has allergies to things and not sure what is causing it. Journaling will help in finding the problems to such things as skin rashes, trouble with sleep or other minor health troubles, all of the symptoms that come with any issue can help in discovering and can help you decide to eliminate those things. When it comes to anything that causes changes good or bad for example: you notice something is causing you not to sleep well after you, eat certain foods, dink certain things, staying up passed a certain time, or that you sleep better when you spend time outdoors, drink only water, or read a book before bed, all is an example of patterns that effect changes in health.

Help in eliminating allergens that aggravate your system: Example: If certain foods or chemicals that aggravate your system and that cause allergy symptoms, such as diarrhea or constipation, mood swings, or other problems, you'll be able to figure out what they are, especially if you are tracking multi-people in your family like your kids, husband or wife. It gives you an easy record to go back and reference when you have a reaction.

You Can Change What You Can't Measure: When I started a workout regime I utilized a journal to tract my success and was able to see areas I needed to work to better improve on. Most professional fitness experts will tell you to journal or keep record of your workouts or any food changes because… you can't change or improve what you can't measure. Journaling will help you get realistic measures of anything your trying to improve upon.

And the Lord answered me: "Write the vision; make it plain on tablets, so he may run who reads it. [46]

---

46 Habakkuk 2:2 (NIV via Biblehub.com)/

CHAPTER 22
First Milk Benefits

• • •

AFTER SEEING MY CHIROPRACTOR AND health doctor, he introduced first milk approach to me. I tried Colostrum-LD (Liposomal Delivery) powder brand and I had some positive reactions such as more energy. It is said that when babies are born, the first mother's milk they ingest helps to protect them against many illnesses. The colostrum, a yellowish liquid, is especially rich in immune factors and high in protein, carbohydrates, and antibodies. Colostrum contains large numbers of antibodies called "secretory immunoglobulin" (IgA) that help protect the mucous membranes in the throat, lungs, and intestines of the infant. Leukocytes are also present in large numbers; these begin protecting the infant from harmful viruses.

Colostrum has been used to treat diarrhea, to improve GI health, to boost the immune system. Colostrum contains immune factors, immunoglobulins, antibodies, proline-rich polypeptides (PRP), lactoferrin, glycoproteins, lactalbumins, cytokines (eg, interleukin, and interferon), growth factors, vitamins, and minerals. There also is a constituent isolated from colostrum that is responsible for uterine and intestinal contraction, and lowering of blood pressure. Ingesting colostrum establishes beneficial bacteria in the digestive tract. There are many different kinds of colostrum on the market.

CHAPTER 23
Health and Sleep

• • •

A GOOD NIGHT'S SLEEP LEADS to good health. It is important that we get enough sleep every day of our lives. If not, it can have a negative effect on everything and can cause a multitude of health problems. For many years, I battled with being able to fall asleep, I took a natural supplement called Kavinace by neuroscience that got me back on a normal sleep pattern. after only taking it for a week I had no problem falling asleep. People often overlook the potential long-term health consequences of insufficient sleep, and the impact that health problems can ultimately have on one's time and productivity. I found this information on sleep to be very interesting, I thought I would share.

If sleep is a problem, it is important to find out what can be done to get the proper sleep. There are two types of sleep, non-REM and REM. Typically, non-REM is 75 percent of our sleep and REM is 25 percent. There are four stages of non-REM sleep before a person reaches REM sleep. After doing some research on sleep stages I found a website to give very detailed information. The website I went to is in the footnote below.[47] There are many people that go to a sleep study facility that will measure your sleep patterns. I have not done this yet, but I know many people that have, and it gave them an understanding on what needed to be done.

---

47 http://www.webmd.com/sleep-disorders/guide/sleep-101, © 2005 - 2017 WebMD, LLC. All rights reserved.

CHAPTER 24

Diacom

• • •

YESTERDAY, I FOUND OUT THAT there is an amazing tool that can analyze your body through the bioelectricity that travels throughout it via the nervous system. I had a Diacom scan done on me after a thermography test, both test went hand in hand and gave the therapist broader information. I recommend that after doing these tests, ask for a printout so you can add it to your journal. This machine reads in a nonlinear fashion as it scans your entire body—all of its organs and organ systems—at the cellular level. It emits electromagnetic waves through the brain stem. The scan uncovers any existing issues your body has and reveals signs of potential issues so that you can take the steps required to prevent or cure the problems. I also found that thermography is similar to thermal imaging

Thermal Imaging is heat detection like the one depicted in the movie Predator. Because our bodies are more or less symmetrical, thermography can be highly effective in detecting abnormalities in paired body parts like limbs or breasts. Full-body thermography scans can be used to keep track of your overall health or monitor progress as you change to a healthier lifestyle. Thermography is also great for monitoring any chronic conditions making sure it's getting better with treatment. Besides early breast cancer detection, thermography can help assess breast cancer risk, which means you can make appropriate lifestyle changes to reduce it. Thermography can be used to detect hormonal imbalances, lymphatic congestion, auto-immune conditions, and much more. If you're interested in this type of procedure, there are clinics that specialize in it. Check in your area for thermography centers.

The Rife Machine

When I went to wellness center near my home, I was introduced to the machine called Rife. The Rife Machine was named after its inventor, Royal Raymond Rife.

Dr. Rife spent his entire life inventing machines that would help people. He envisioned and tested a machine that would destroy pathogens, bacteria, and even viruses with no toxic side effects. He theorized that the same device could eradicate cancer by altering the cancer's cellular environment or by killing cancer viruses with an electronic or ultrasonic beam

The Rife machine uses a variable frequency, pulsed radio transmitter to produce mechanical resonance within the cells of the physical body. Rife machines work on the principle of sympathetic resonance, which states that if there are two similar objects and one of them is vibrating, the other will begin to vibrate as well, even if they are not touching. In the same way that a sound wave can induce resonance in a crystal glass and ultrasound can be used to destroy gallstones, Dr. Rife's instrument uses sympathetic resonance to physically vibrate the cells of the parasite resulting in possible elimination. Vibration between two objects can be seen in everyday life, from a tuning fork to a guitar string. The destructive capabilities of resonance have been widely demonstrated, for example when an opera singer hits a particular note and breaks a glass. In this instance the musical tone sets the glass in motion, and as the motion builds the glass shatters. The pulsed wave used in the Rife system produces a mechanical vibration, whereby the low amplitude input leads to a large amplitude vibration in the target. If the induced resonant vibration is intense enough, the target cell, tissue, or molecule will be destroyed.

CHAPTER 25
Breath of Air

• • •

THE QUALITY OF THE AIR we all breathe is essential to good health. Unfortunately, good quality air is compromised in many different ways. Inside your home, alone, you can breathe in pathogens and chemical components from building materials, molds, dust mites, fumes from cleaners, insect repellants, and fumes from fabrics like those in draperies, clothing, and furniture. Other things include pet dander, human dander, and cigarette smoke.

This is where I started my research into my illness. I had begun testing the air coming from the ducts in the central air-conditioning system in my home. My pasture had purchased a mold kit from the local Home Depot for me and, sure enough, mold was present somewhere in the air ducts. This test took a total of four days to complete, and when the test came out positive, I knew this was a factor in trigger-ing my illness. A few years earlier, I had undergone allergy testing and discovered that I was allergic to mold. We are exposed to all

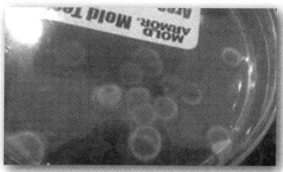

Figure 10 "Mold" Armor mold test kit

types of molds indoors and outdoors. Molds produce allergens, irritants and, sometimes toxins that can cause adverse reactions in humans depending on the length of exposure, age, allergies and sensitivities that person may have. The normal reactions for sensitive people would be a runny nose, sneezing, nasal congestion, watery eyes, skin rashes, and itching. In rare instances, people may develop pneumonia. People with a weakened immune system, such as those who are immune-compromised or immune-suppressed from drug treatment, can contract infectious diseases from mold. Such infections can affect the skin, eyes, lungs, or some organs. Another source of irritation from mold exposure comes from substances known as microbial volatile organic compounds (mVOCs[48]). These compounds are produced through fungal metabolism and are released directly into the air, often giving off strong or unpleasant odors. Exposure to mVOCs from molds can irritate the eyes and respiratory system and has been linked to symptoms such as headaches, dizziness, fatigue, nasal irritation and nausea. The effects of mVOCs are not completely understood and research is still in the early stages. These are considered opportunistic infections that usually do not affect healthy people. Mycotoxins, are potent substances produced by some molds. People can be exposed to mycotoxins through inhalation, ingestion or skin contact. Many molds, including species commonly found indoors, are capable of producing mycotoxins.

If you're interested in an affordable clean-air purifier, check out the products at austinair.com. The company sells all types of air purifiers for home and office.

---

48 Microbial Volatile Organic Compound (mVOCs)

CHAPTER 26
Blood Work and Testing

• • •

MANY DIFFERENT TYPES OF BLOOD tests can be performed these days. Documenting the changes in your health from year to year in your health journal can form the backbone of a good disease-prevention program. For this, start with basic tests that will give you a snapshot of your overall health and serve as a baseline for detecting changes. If you want to do any blood work from home, there are many online companies that offer in home blood test kits, going this route, you need to research and do your homework in finding the right company, due to a lot of them giving inaccurate or bogus test results. Also, there are many any lab test now facilities you could research and find one that carries the test you're looking for. Below are some basic tests and a list of the elements to monitor:

Complete Blood Count (CBC)—This test provides a broad range of diagnostic information to assess your vascular, liver, kidney, and blood cell status. The Complete Blood Count measures the number, variety, percentage, concentration, and quality of platelets, red blood cells, and white blood cells, and thus is useful in screening for infections, anemias, and other hematological abnormalities.

High-density lipoprotein (HDL)—This is a lipoprotein with a relatively high concentration of protein and low concentration of lipids that incorporates cholesterol and transports it to the liver. High levels are associated with a decreased risk of atherosclerosis and coronary artery disease also, called HDL cholesterol.

Low-density lipoprotein (LDL)—This is a lipoprotein with a relatively high concentration of lipids and low concentration of protein that incorporates cholesterol and transports it to cells. High levels are associated with an increased risk of atherosclerosis and coronary artery disease. It is also called LDL cholesterol.

Triglycerides—Fatty compounds synthesized from carbohydrates during the process of digestion and stored in the body's adipose (fat) tissues. High levels of triglycerides in the blood are associated with insulin resistance.

Cholesterol—a steroid alcohol found in animal fats and oils, bile, blood, brain tissue, milk, egg yolk, myelin sheaths of nerve fibers, liver, kidneys, and adrenal glands. It is a precursor of bile acids and steroid hormones, and it occurs in the most common type of gallstone, in atheroma of the arteries, in various cysts, and in carcinomatous tissue. Most of the body's cholesterol is synthesized by the liver, but some is obtained in the diet from animal-derived foods. Plant-derived foods are cholesterol-free. Cholesterol is not transported free in the blood but is bound to certain proteins to form lipoproteins. Two important fractions of the serum lipoproteins are high-density lipoproteins (HDL) and low-density lipoproteins (LDL). High levels of total serum cholesterol have been shown to be associated with a high risk for coronary artery disease and myocardial infarction. Research has drawn a distinction between HDL-C, the cholesterol carried on high-density lipoproteins and LDL-C, the cholesterol carried on low-density lipoproteins. The balance between HDL-C and LDL-C is more significant than the total concentration of cholesterol in the blood. The risk of coronary heart disease increases as LDL-C increases and HDL-C decreases.

Glucose—a six-carbon aldose occurring as the d- form and found as a free monosaccharide in fruits and other plants or combined in glucosides and di-, oligo-, and polysaccharides. It is the end product of carbohydrate metabolism, and is the chief source of energy for living organisms, its utilization being controlled by insulin. Excess glucose is converted to glycogen and stored in the liver and muscles for use as needed and, beyond that, is converted to fat and stored as adipose tissue. Glucose appears in the urine in diabetes mellitus. In pharmaceuticals, called dextrose.

Fibrinogen—a high-molecular-weight protein in the blood plasma that by the action of thrombin is converted into fibrin; called also factor i. In the clotting mechanism, fibrin threads form a meshwork for the basis of a blood clot. Most of the fibrinogen in the circulating blood is formed in the liver. Normal quantities of fibrinogen in the plasma vary from 100 to 700 mg per 100 ml of plasma. Commercial preparations of human fibrinogen are used to restore blood fibrinogen levels to normal after extensive surgery, or to treat diseases and hemorrhagic conditions that are complicated by afibrinogenemia.

Hemoglobin A1C—an allosteric protein found in erythrocytes that transports molecular oxygen (O2) in the blood. Symbol Hb.

Oxygenated hemoglobin (oxyhemoglobin) is bright red in color; hemoglobin unbound to oxygen (deoxyhemoglobin) is darker. This accounts for the bright red color of arterial blood, in which the hemoglobin is about 97% saturated with oxygen. Venous blood is darker because it is only about 20–70% saturated, depending on how much oxygen is being used by the tissues. The affinity of hemoglobin for carbon monoxide is 210 times as strong as its affinity for oxygen. The complex formed (carboxyhemoglobin) cannot transport oxygen. Thus, carbon monoxide poisoning results in hypoxia and asphyxiation. Another form of hemoglobin that cannot transport oxygen is methemoglobin, in which the iron atom is oxidized to the +3 oxidation state. During the life span of a red cell, hemoglobin is slowly oxidized to methemoglobin. At least four different enzyme systems can convert methemoglobin back to hemoglobin. When these are defective or overloaded, methemoglobinemia[49], in which high methemoglobin levels cause dyspnea and cyanosis, may result. As red cells wear out or are damaged, they are ingested by macrophages of the reticuloendothelial system. The porphyrin ring of heme is converted to the bile pigment bilirubin, which is excreted by the liver. [50]The iron is transported to the bone marrow to be incorporated in the hemoglobin of newly formed erythrocytes. This test measures a person's blood sugar control over the last two to three months and is an independent predictor of heart disease risk in persons with or without diabetes. Maintaining healthy hemoglobin A1C levels may also help patients with diabetes to prevent some of the complications of the disease.

Dehydroepiandrosterone (DHEA)—a steroid secreted chiefly by the adrenal cortex, but also by the testis; it is the principal precursor of urinary 17-ketosteroids. Weakly androgenic itself, it is metabolized to δ-5 androstenediol, a hormone with both androgenic and estrogenic effects, and is one of the precursors of testosterone. Serum levels are elevated in adrenal virilism. It may function as a neurotransmitter. DHEA secretion begins during fetal life, reaches a peak in the third decade, and declines steadily thereafter; the level at age eighty is only 10–20 percent of the peak level. This decline has been speculatively associated with the changes of aging. Commercial formulations of DHEA are marketed as dietary supplements, although this substance is neither a nutrient nor a component of the human food chain. DHEA has been promoted for the prevention of degenerative diseases including atherosclerosis, Alzheimer dementia, Parkinsonism, and other effects of aging. None of the alleged

---

49 Methemoglobinemia is a condition caused by elevated levels of methemoglobin in the blood, https://en.wikipedia.org/wiki/Methemoglobinemia, 22 July 2017, at 23:56.

50   http://medical-dictionary.thefreedictionary.com/hemoglobin+A+1c

benefits has been demonstrated in large, randomized clinical trials. Limited studies in animals and human subjects suggest that DHEA reduces the percentage of body fat, perhaps by blocking the storage of energy as fat. Long-term administration to postmenopausal women has been associated with insulin resistance, hypertension, and reduction of LDL cholesterol levels. An analysis of 16 preparations of DHEA by high-performance liquid chromatography showed a variation in content from 0 to150 percent of the labeled strength; only seven products fell between the expected 90 to 110 percent of labeled strength.

Prostate—a gland in the male that surrounds the bladder NECK and URETHRA; it consists of a median lobe and two lateral lobes and is made up partly of glandular matter (whose ducts empty into the prostatic portion of the urethra) and partly of muscular fibers that encircle the urethra. It contributes to the seminal fluid a secretion containing acid phosphatase, citric acid, and proteolytic enzymes, which account for the liquefaction of the coagulated semen. The rate of secretion increases greatly during sexual stimulation. Enlargement of the prostate (benign prostatic hypertrophy) is a common complaint in men over 50 years of age. Because of its position around the urethra, enlargement of the prostate quickly interferes with the normal passage of urine from the bladder. Urination becomes increasingly difficult, and the bladder never feels completely emptied. If the condition is left untreated, continued enlargement of the prostate eventually obstructs the urethra completely, and emergency measures become necessary to empty the bladder. If the prostate is markedly enlarged, chronic constipation may result. The usual remedy is prostatectomy. In men, over the age of 60, cancer of the prostate is common these days. Prostatitis is a relatively common inflammation of the prostate and may be acute or chronic.

Homocysteine—Homocysteine is a sulfur-containing amino acid that occurs naturally in all humans. It is broken down in the body through two metabolic pathways. The chemical changes that must occur to break down homocysteine require the presence of folic acid (also called folate) and vitamins B6 and B12. The level of homocysteine in the blood is influenced by the presence of these substances. Homocysteine is a rare genetic disorder that occurs in about one in every 200,000 individuals. This congenital metabolic disorder causes large amounts of homocystinuria[51] to be excreted in the urine. Homocystinuria is associated mental retardation and the development of heart disease before age 30. In the late 1960s, doctors documented that individuals with homocystinuria developed narrowing of the arteries at a very early age, sometimes even in childhood. Although homocystinuria is rare, this finding stimulated research on whether people who did not have homocystinuria but who did have unusually high levels of homocysteine in their blood were at greater risk of developing heart disease or stroke. Many risk factors, including family history of heart disease, smoking, obesity, lack of exercise, diabetes, high levels of low-density lipoprotein cholesterol (LDL or "bad" cholesterol), low levels of high-density lipoprotein cholesterol (HDL or "good" cholesterol), and high blood pressure have been documented to increase the risk of stroke and heart disease. With so many other risk factors, it has been difficult to determine whether high levels of homocysteine are an independent risk factor for the development these diseases. However, a substantial number of controlled, well-designed, and well-documented studies have shown that individuals who have high levels of homocysteine in the blood are at increased risk of developing blocked blood vessels, a condition known as occlusive arterial disease or at risk to worsen atherosclerosis ("hardening of the arteries"). From 2000 to 2010, studies also suggested that high levels of homocysteine were associated with poorer

---

[51] Homocystinuria is an inherited disorder in which the body is unable to process certain building blocks of proteins properly. https://ghr.nlm.nih.gov/condition/homocystinuria/ October 3rd 2017

mental functioning, leading to ongoing investigations into the role of homocysteine in Alzheimer's disease. Additional studies have also suggested that high levels of homocysteine can lead to osteoporosis and an increased risk of broken bones in the elderly.

In Japan, increased homocysteine levels were found to be associated with the presence of gallstones in middle-aged men. Investigators suggested that this association "may partly explain the reported high prevalence rate of coronary heart disease" in persons with gallstones. A study from the Netherlands has shown that among normal individuals aged 30–80, elevated homocysteine concentrations are associated with prolonged lower cognitive performance. Natural therapies may help to optimize homocysteine levels. You may wish to discuss with your doctor, the use of vitamin B12, vitamin B6, folic acid, and trimethyl glycine.

C-Reactive Proteins—C-reactive protein is not normally found in the blood of healthy people. It appears after an injury, infection, or inflammation and disappears when the injury heals or the infection or inflammation goes away. Research suggests that patients with prolonged elevated levels of C-reactive protein are at an increased risk for heart disease, stroke, hypertension (high blood pressure), diabetes, and metabolic syndrome (insulin resistance, a precursor of type 2 diabetes). The amount of CRP produced by the body varies from person to person, and this difference is affected by an individual's genetic makeup (accounting for almost half of the variation in CRP levels between different people) and lifestyle. Higher CRP levels tend to be found in individuals who smoke, have high blood pressure, are overweight and do not exercise, whereas lean, athletic individuals tend to have lower CRP levels. The research shows that too much inflammation can sometimes have adverse effects on the blood vessels which transport oxygen and nutrients throughout the body. Atherosclerosis, which involves the formation of fatty deposits or plaques in the inner walls of the arteries, is now considered in many ways an inflammatory disorder of the blood vessels, similar to the way arthritis can be considered an inflammatory disorder of the bones and joints. Inflammation affects the atherosclerotic phase of heart disease and can cause plaques to rupture, which produces a clot and interfere with blood flow, causing a heart attack or stroke. There is an association between elevated levels of inflammatory markers (including CRP) and the future development of heart disease. This correlation applies even to apparently healthy men and women who have normal cholesterol levels. CRP level can be used by physicians as part of the assessment of a patient's risk for heart disease because it is a stable molecule and can be easily measured with a simple blood test. In patients already suffering from heart disease, doctors can use CRP levels to determine which patients are at high risk for recurring coronary events. Normal range for C-Reactive Protein for a female is 0-3 mg/L optimum range for men is <0.55 mg/L.

Thyroid Stimulating Hormone (TSH)—Secreted by the pituitary gland, thyroid stimulating hormone (TSH) controls thyroid hormone secretion in the thyroid. When blood levels fall below normal, this indicates hyperthyroidism (increased thyroid activity, also called thyrotoxicosis), and when values are above normal, this suggests hypothyroidism (low thyroid activity). Overt hyper- or hypothyroidism is Because the symptoms of thyroid imbalance may be nonspecific or absent and may progress slowly, and since many doctors do not routinely screen for thyroid function, people with mild hyper- or hypothyroidism can go undiagnosed for some time. Undiagnosed mild disease can progress to clinical disease states. This is a dangerous scenario, since people with hypothyroidism and elevated serum cholesterol and LDL have an increased risk of atherosclerosis. Mild hypothyroidism (low thyroid gland function) may be associated with reversible hypercholesterolemia (high blood cholesterol) and cognitive dysfunction, as well as such nonspecific symptoms as fatigue, depression, cold intolerance, dry skin, constipation, and weight gain. Mild hyperthyroidism is often associated with atrial fibrillation (a disturbance of heart rhythm), reduced bone mineral density, and nonspecific symptoms such as fatigue, weight loss, heat intolerance, nervousness, insomnia, muscle weakness, shortness of breath, and heart palpitations. Generally easy to diagnose, but subclinical disease can be more elusive.

To dive deeper into your health status, consider these tests.

Immunoglobulin M (IgM)—This is a basic antibody that is present in B cells. IgM antibodies appear early in the course of an infection and usually reappear to a less extent after further exposure.

IgM in normal serum is often found to bind to specific pathogens, even in the absence of prior immunization.

Immunoglobulin E (IgE)—IgE may be elevated in an allergic patient. IgE are antibodies produced by the immune system. If you have an allergy, your immune system overreacts to an allergen by producing antibodies. These antibodies travel to cells that release chemicals, causing an allergic reaction. This reaction usually causes symptoms in the nose, lungs, throat, or on the skin. Each type of IgE has specific "radar" for each type of allergen. That's why some people are only allergic to cat dander (they only have the IgE antibodies specific to cat dander); while others have allergic reactions to multiple allergens because they have many more types of IgE antibodies.

Immunoglobulin A (IgA)—IgA serves as a neutralizing antibody preventing invading pathogens by attaching and penetrating epithelial surfaces. It plays a critical role in mucosal immunity such as found in the nose, rectum, ears, mouth, and vaginal area. More IgA is produced in mucosal linings than all the other types of antibodies combined. It provides protection against microbes that multiply in body secretions. IgA is very weak complement activating antibody. Patients suffering from selective Immunoglobulin A (IgA) deficiency can have normal levels of the other antibodies, fully functioning T-cells, phagocytes, and other components of the immune system. Patients who suffer from a selective IgA deficiency are more prone to autoimmune disorders like Rheumatoid Arthritis, Lupus, allergies and asthma.

Antinuclear Antibodies (ANA)—This is an antibody showing an affinity for nuclear antigens including DNA and found in the serum of a high proportion of patients with systemic lupus erythematosus, rheumatoid arthritis, and certain collagen diseases, and in some of their healthy relatives; as well as about 1% of otherwise healthy people. Different antinuclear antibodies generate distinctive patterns on immunofluorescence staining tests. These patterns have clinical relevance and reflect which nuclear constituents (autoantigens) are generative specific antibody responses. Currently my ANA is abnormally high, I believe this just means my body is dealing with abnormally high inflammation.

FINAL THOUGHTS

● ● ●

Disease and illness are on the rise, but they do not have to take our lives from us. We can choose to take accountability for our own health and do the research ourselves. You will be surprised what you will find and learn. Take ownership now. Start a health journal. If you go to see the physician, ask a lot of questions and then document the responses. If you have a religion, pray daily.

Make better choices to better your health. Write down the things you eat and do that are good, and then write down the things you question. For example, do I smoke or eat a lot of junk food? Do I eat too much red meat and dairy products? Ask yourself whether you can live without those things or replace them with better choices. Try to move to a more chemical free diet, get the whole family involved by going to a local farm and picking your own produce. If you enjoy gardening, build your own vegetable garden by following an organic way.

Learn your body inside and out, and write everything in your journal. Note moles that look questionable. Be in tune to all the signals that your body is sending. Ask yourself whether the pain you feel is present all the time. Does it radiate?

Don't be afraid to examine the color of your poop and pee. Know that researching can be helpful in finding some answers—answers that will get you closer to the root cause of an ailment. Then you can either tackle it through proper medication or through natural means that will put you on the path to healing yourself.

As I look around, more and more people have some type of disease or illness, and new types are showing up every year. I cannot even count how many types illness there are.

I wrote this book to inspire others to take control and accountability for their own health. I have always wanted to see people well and able to enjoy life. Research is a great way to begin finding answers to your health concerns. Seek physicians whose true passion is helping people get back to a healthy, happy life. I recommend doing annual blood testing to add information to your health journal. As you age, you will be able to see changes and potentially prevent life-threatening diseases. There are tons of physicians who want to see their patients healthy and happy.

I ultimately recommend having God in your life. Give it all to God. Keep faith in Him. He is our hope. Pray always. Keep stress under control. Eat right, and get enough sleep. Find someone you can talk to—don't keep things bottled up. Live and love life; it all has a happy ending.

I hope this book inspires all who read it, and contained helpful information. This is my first book; I have learned a great deal by my own journey, researching and sharing these topics. Disease, virtually ALL disease, begins as a Spiritual problem. It begins in the "heart" because we want to live, eat, think, act, and handle stress our own way, rather than GOD'S way. We are in rebellion against God, whether we realize and acknowledge it or not. Only much later do the physical symptoms appear, and as a result consequences.

Research Me

We believe we have Free Will and the right to exercise it, but Jesus said, "I came NOT to do My OWN will, but the WILL of Him who sent Me."[52]

The one thing I always remind myself, family, and children is to always follow your heart, to live life by God's commandments, because when we don't the things we want in life, will not come easy, only because God is trying to keep us on the path of righteousness.

Father God, thank you for the life you have given me and the gift you give all of us, for giving us the patience we need, for giving us hope in the answer you will provide, and for sending your son Jesus to give us a new life, starting at the cross. We love and thank you. In Jesus's mighty name, amen!

---

52 john 6:38 (NIV via blueletterbible.org)

ACKNOWLEDGMENTS

• • •

I THANK MY HUSBAND FOR always being supportive and lifting my spirits each and every day and helping with this process. To both of my children, my mom, dad, and sisters, thank you for believing in me and thank you to twin sister for providing all the art work in this manuscript. Thank you to the pastors from Air1 radio for praying with me and Pastor Glenn Feehan of True North Frisco, Texas. Thank you, Jesus, for filling my heart with words needed to express in this endeavor, and helping me with strength, faith, peace, and love through this health journey, it was an exciting experience writing my first book.

AUTHOR BIOGRAPHY

• • •

SINDY P. HEARD WAS BORN in Baton Rouge, Louisiana, in 1968, one of a pair of identical twins. Since her parents' work required frequent relocation, Sindy lived in various towns in the southern United States, mostly in Florida and Texas. She now calls North Texas her home. Sindy has always enjoyed exploring new places and has traveled internationally, living in Switzerland before marrying. She has two children, is a certified scuba diver, and loves animals. At the age of twenty-eight, she started noticing the first signs of Friedreich's ataxia and has worked tirelessly since then to find a cure. On this journey, she has learned more about her God, her body, and her illness. One thing she has discovered is that people do not take full accountability for their own health and well-being. In this book, readers will find a roadmap and a blueprint showing the steps each person must consider for strengthening and protecting his or her own health.

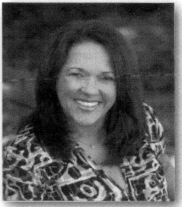

Figure 11 Sindy P. Heard 2016

Isaiah 40:31
But those who wait for the Lord's help find renewed strength; they rise up as if they had eagles' wings, they run without growing weary, they walk without getting tired.

PERSONAL JOURNAL

• • •

NOTE: INFORMATION YOU CAN TRACK around your health helps your discovery.

Date	Entry

Made in the USA
Columbia, SC
15 January 2018